Practical Manual of Cardiology

Annapoorna Kini • Samin Sharma
Jagat Narula
Editors

Practical Manual of Interventional Cardiology

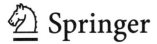 Springer

Editors
Annapoorna Kini, MD, MRCP, FACC
Mount Sinai School of Medicine
New York, NY
USA

Jagat Narula
Mount Sinai School of Medicine
New York, NY
USA

Samin Sharma, MD, FACC
Mount Sinai School of Medicine
New York, NY
USA

ISBN 978-1-4471-6580-4   ISBN 978-1-4471-6581-1   (eBook)
DOI 10.1007/978-1-4471-6581-1
Springer London Heidelberg New York Dordrecht

Library of Congress Control Number: 2014957170

Springer is part of Springer Science+Business Media (www.springer.com)

Preface

Since the introduction of balloon angioplasty by Andreas Gruentzig in 1977, interventional cardiology has immensely proliferated in the last 37 years. Various new interventional devices and modifications of existing interventional techniques have improved the safety and long-term benefits of the interventional procedures. From the Cardiovascular Catheterization Lab of Mount Sinai Heart at Mount Sinai Hospital, we have compiled all commonly used interventional devices and their appropriate step-by-step technique of use in this manual of Interventional Cardiology. This is a step-by-step approach to master class in interventional techniques. The main focus of this book is to educate and prepare the interventional fellows in their day-to-day practice with an ultimate goal of making them safe and confident operators. We are indebted to all the authors, especially our interventional fellows of 2013–2014, who have made possible this master class manual.

New York, NY, USA
Annapoorna Kini, MD, MRCP, FACC
Samin Sharma, MD, FACC
Jagat Narula

Contents

Contributors

Leslie Innasimuthu, MD Department of Interventional Cardiology, Mount Sinai Hospital, New York, NY, USA

Annapoorna Kini, MD, MRCP, FACC Department of Interventional Cardiology, Mount Sinai Hospital, New York, NY, USA

Mayur Lakhani, MD Department of Interventional Cardiology, Mount Sinai Hospital, New York, NY, USA

Surabhi Madhwal, MD Department of Interventional Cardiology, Mount Sinai Hospital, New York, NY, USA

Ajith Nair, MD Department of Interventional Cardiology, Mount Sinai Hospital, New York, NY, USA

Sadhik Raja Panwar, MD Department of Interventional Cardiology, Mount Sinai Hospital, New York, NY, USA

Rikesh Patel, MD Department of Interventional Cardiology, Mount Sinai Hospital, New York, NY, USA

Robert Pyo, MD Department of Interventional Cardiology, Mount Sinai Hospital, New York, NY, USA

Anitha Rajamanickam, MD Department of Interventional Cardiology, Mount Sinai Hospital, New York, NY, USA

Ravinder Singh Rao, MD Department of Interventional Cardiology, Mount Sinai Hospital, New York, NY, USA

Rahul Sawant, MD Department of Interventional Cardiology, Mount Sinai Hospital, New York, NY, USA

Nagendra Boopathy Senguttuvan, MD, DM Department of Interventional Cardiology, Mount Sinai Hospital, New York, NY, USA

Samin Sharma, MD, FACC Department of Interventional Cardiology, Mount Sinai Hospital, New York, NY, USA

Joseph Sweeny, MD Department of Interventional Cardiology,
Mount Sinai Hospital, New York, NY, USA

Faramarz (Taj) Tehrani, MD Department of Interventional Cardiology,
Mount Sinai Hospital, New York, NY, USA

Christopher J. Varughese, MD Department of Interventional Cardiology,
Mount Sinai Hospital, New York, NY, USA

Part I

Interventional Basics

Basics of Radiation Safety

1

Ravinder Singh Rao, Anitha Rajamanickam,
and Joseph Sweeny

Introduction

Cardiac catheterization procedures expose both the patient and operator to the hazards of radiation. The hazards of repeated radiation exposure are serious, but not obvious. Four rational principles are evident.

- Radiation-induced biological effects are the result of random statistical probability for low radiation doses. The probability of these effects is directly proportional to the radiation dose received. The effects of radiation are described in Fig. 1.1.
- Since radiation-induced biological effects are random, and no threshold dose exists for these effects, even a small dose could potentially induce biological effects, and therefore no level of radiation exposure can be considered completely safe.
- Radiation exposure is cumulative and there is no washout phenomenon as with other toxin exposures.
- Each person involved in the cardiac catheterization lab has accepted a certain degree of risk posed by radiation exposure. Current regulatory considerations for radiation limit are listed in Table 1.1.

R.S. Rao, MD • A. Rajamanickam, MD • J. Sweeny, MD (✉)
Department of Interventional Cardiology, Mount Sinai Hospital,
One Gustave Levy Place, Madison Avenue, New York, NY 10029, USA
e-mail: drravindersinghrao@yahoo.co.in; arajamanickam@gmail.com,
Anitha.rajamanickam@mountsinai.org; Joseph.sweeny@mountsinai.org

© Springer-Verlag London 2014
A. Kini et al. (eds.), *Practical Manual of Interventional Cardiology*,
DOI 10.1007/978-1-4471-6581-1_1

Fig. 1.1 Effects of radiation

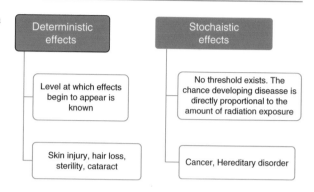

Table 1.1 Current regulatory considerations for radiation limit

Tissue	Risk	Recommended maximum dose	
		NCRP	ICRP
Occupational	Stochastic	50 mSv/year	100 mSv/5 year
Lens of the eye	Stochastic	150 mSv/year	150 mSv/year
Extremities	Stochastic	500 mSv/year	500 mSv/year
Embryo-fetus	Stochastic	0.5 mSv/month	1 mSv/term
General public	Stochastic	1 mSv/year	1 mSv/year

National Council on Radiation Protection and Measurements (NCRP)
International Commission on Radiological Protection (ICRP)
10 mSv = 1 rem

ALARA

ALARA is a radiation safety principle and regulatory requirement for radiation safety of all personnel. It stands for "as low as reasonably achievable." If the radiation exposure exceeds the ALARA limit, the radiation safety officer (RSO) will have a discussion with operator to assess different possibility of radiation exposure reduction and regarding the possible side effects. Three principles help in maintaining ALARA practice:

- *Time*: Reducing the duration of radiation exposure will reduce the dose.
- *Distance*: Radiation follows the inverse square law. Doubling the distance from source will reduce the radiation exposure by factor of 4.
- *Shielding*: Using absorbent material like lead for x-rays reduces the exposure.

Monitoring Patient Dose

Fluoroscopic time: Total time of fluoroscopy use during procedure.
Air kerma (AK): Refers to x-ray energy delivered to air at the interventional reference point. It is a measure of patient's dose burden and correlates to determine the effects.

Dose area product (DAP)/air kerma-area product: Product of total radiation dose and area of x-ray field. It is expressed as Gy.cm^2. It is a measure of radiation exposure and correlates with possible risk of stochastic effects.

Safety Components

Radiation monitoring

- Mandate the use of the dosimeter.
- Review the practice pattern of every individual and especially if the dosimeter records high radiation doses.
- Advisory agencies such as NCRP give 2 options of measuring effective dose equivalent (EDE) for workers who use lead aprons. The first option is to have one badge on the collar outside the apron and the other badge under the apron at the waist level. The second option is to use only one badge outside the lead apron on the collar level.

Shielding

- Lead garments to protect the gonads and approximately 80 % of the bone marrow.
- 0.5 mm lead apron stops approximately 95 % of the scatter radiation.
- Separate thyroid collars, especially for the young and in those whose radiation dose exceeds 4 mSv/month.
- 0.25 mm lead eyeglasses for eye protection (radiation can cause posterior sub-capsular cataracts).
- Use of below the table-mounted shields.
- Transparent ceiling-mounted shields.
- Disposable radiation absorbing sterile drapes.
- Proper maintenance and periodic inspection (atleast once a year) of lead aprons.

Procedural Issues [1]

Precautions to minimize exposure to patient and operator

- Utilize radiation only when imaging is necessary to support clinical care.
- Minimize use of cine.
- Minimize use of steep angles.
- Minimize use of magnification modes.
- Minimize frame rate of fluoroscopy and cine.
- Keep the image intensifier close to the patient.
- Utilize collimation to the fullest extent as possible.
- Monitor radiation dose in real time.

Precautions to minimize operator exposure

- Use and maintain appropriate protective garments.
- Maximize distance of operator from x-ray source and patient.
- Keep above and below table shields in proper position at all times.
- Keep all body parts out of field.

Precautions to minimize patient exposure

- Keep table height as high as comfortable for the operator.
- Vary the imaging beam angle to minimize exposure to any one skin area.
- Keep patient's extremities out of beam.

Impact on Patient Care

Inclusion of radiation dose on cardiac catheterization reports is mandatory.
Follow-up based on AK:

- AK >5 Gy:
  - Patient education regarding potential skin changes like redness and report if seen.
  - Patient to be contacted within 30 days.
- AK >10 Gy:
  - Qualified physicist to perform detailed analysis and calculate peak skin dose
  - Office visit in 2–4 weeks with skin examination
- PSD (peak skin dose) >15 Gy:
  - Contact hospital risk management.
  - Notification to regulatory agencies.

Reference

1. Chambers CE, Fetterly KA, Holzer R, Lin PJ, Blankenship JC, Balter S, Laskey WK. Radiation safety program for the cardiac catheterization laboratory. Catheter Cardiovasc Interv. 2011;77(4):546–56. doi:10.1002/ccd.22867. PubMed PMID: 21254324.

Achieving Perfect Vascular Access

2

Anitha Rajamanickam and Robert Pyo

The femoral artery is the most commonly used arterial site of access in the United States (>90 % in 2011). The radial artery access is currently gaining popularity [1]. The brachial artery, axillary artery, ulnar artery, and femoral artery cutdown for access are rarely used now.

Femoral Artery

Obtaining optimal femoral artery access is crucial for procedural and clinical success and still remains one of the crucial technical challenges for the interventional cardiologist. Access site complications remains an important cause of cardiac catheterization morbidity and mortality. A "high" sheath insertion above the inguinal ligament increases the risk of retroperitoneal bleeding, while a "low" sheath insertion into the profunda femoris or the superficial femoral artery (SFA) may result in arteriovenous fistula, pseudoaneurysm, or limb ischemia.

Contraindications for femoral artery access

- Femoral access: Not performed in INR ≥2.5 [3].
- Venous access: Not performed in INR ≥4.
- If a percutaneous procedure needs to be performed urgently on a patient taking warfarin, periprocedural correction of coagulopathy needs to be instituted rapidly with 1–2 units of fresh frozen plasma (FFP) if anticoagulation can be reversed

A. Rajamanickam, MD (✉) • R. Pyo, MD
Department of Interventional Cardiology, Mount Sinai Hospital,
One Gustave Levy Place, Madison Avenue, New York, NY 10029, USA
e-mail: arajamanickam@gmail.com, Anitha.rajamanickam@mountsinai.org;
Robert.pyo@mountsinai.org

© Springer-Verlag London 2014
A. Kini et al. (eds.), *Practical Manual of Interventional Cardiology*,
DOI 10.1007/978-1-4471-6581-1_2

Table 2.1 Femoral sheath size by procedure

Procedure		Sheath size
Diagnostic cardiac catheterization		5 Fr
PCI – most PCIs including orbital atherectomy and rotational atherectomy burr <2 mm		6 Fr
PCI with planned two-stent strategy for bifurcation lesions [modified T technique, SKS technique, V technique] or rotational atherectomy burr of 2 mm		7 Fr
Rotational atherectomy burr of 2.15 mm or 2.25 mm		8 Fr
Balloon aortic valvuloplasty	18 mm balloon	10 Fr
	20 mm balloon	11 Fr
	22 mm balloon	12 Fr
	23–25 mm balloon	13 Fr
Impella	2.5	13 Fr
	CS	14 Fr
Transcatheter aortic valve replacement	Core valve	18 Fr
	Edwards SAPIEN valve	22–24 Fr

safely. In patients at a very high risk of thromboembolism, bridge with unfractionated heparin or low molecular weight heparin.

- Avoid in morbid obesity, severe peripheral vascular disease, or aortic dissection. Can use old synthetic grafts for puncture if necessary.
- Avoid in patients on factor Xa inhibitors (rivaroxaban, apixaban) and direct thrombin inhibitor (dabigatran) unless the patients have been off these agents for 24–48 h. [4].

Sheath selection Five French(Fr) sheath and catheters will suffice for most diagnostic cardiac catheterizations. The common femoral artery [CFA] diameter in women and diabetics tends to be smaller, and therefore a smaller sheath may be selected [5]. The sheath can be upsized as needed for interventions (see Table 2.1).

Pearls
- In obese patients tape the pannus to stretch the skin tightly over the femoral head.
- Use long sheaths 25 or 45 cm in patients with tortuous peripheral arteries

Needle used High-risk patients may require the assist of a micropuncture needle for a more controlled access into the common femoral artery so that a vascular closure device may be employed to close the access site after the procedure.

These patients include:
- Extremely obese patients with deep vasculature.
- Patients who are anticoagulated or have a coagulopathy.
- Patients with known or suspected peripheral arterial disease may require arterial access into a relatively non-diseased portion of the vessel.

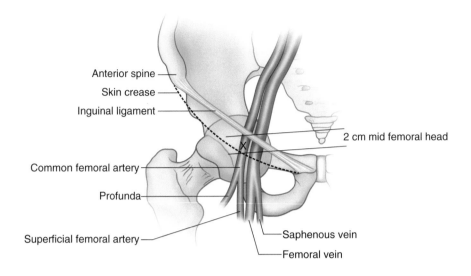

Fig. 2.1 Perfect location for femoral access

Perfect access location

- The segment of the common femoral artery below the inguinal ligament [1–2 cm below the line traced from the anterosuperior iliac spine to the pubic tubercle] is the ideal location for arterial access. This correlates roughly to an area that is at the mid third of the femoral head which is usually above the femoral bifurcation and below the lowest point of the course of the inferior epigastric artery (Fig. 2.1).
- Femoral artery bifurcation is below the inferior border of the femoral head in 80 % of cases and below the inguinal ligament and middle of the femoral head in 100 % of cases. The femoral artery lies on the medial third of the femoral head in 92 % of patients and only 8 % have the arterial completely medial to the femoral head [6–8].

> **Pearl**
> - The inguinal crease is not a reliable landmark [9]. However, in general, we have found it safer not to puncture above the inguinal crease.

Common steps for both micropuncture and regular access needle

- Fluoro the femoral head with an overlying hemostat to mark the bottom border of the femoral head and palpate the point of maximal pulsation at this level. Aim for an area between the lower borders of the femoral head to the mid femoral head (Fig. 2.1). The needle entry point at the skin level should be at the lower border of the femoral head.

- Lidocaine: Generous 20–30 cc infiltration of the skin. Create a subcutaneous wheal at the entry site with 3–4 cc of lidocaine and then gradually deliver an additional 16–27 cc of local anesthetic to the deeper subcutaneous tissue covering the anticipated needle path from the skin to the arterial. Monitor the ECG for bradycardia and the patient for any vagal reaction.
- After a small skin nick, the subcutaneous space can be opened gently, with blunt forceps. This provides a pathway for blood to ooze out of the skin in case of bleeding and allows for early identification of complications (this step may be considered when Perclose™ technique of closure is planned, especially for closure of large sheaths).
- Enter the front wall of the arterial. Advance either the 18 gauge needle or the micropuncture needle at a 45° angle until backflow of the arterial blood is noted at the needle hub (Fig. 2.2. Step Ia). Advancing the needle at more vertical angle could result in kinking of the sheath and using a more horizontal angle may result in a high stick. Note that the backflow of blood when an 18 gauge needle is used should be brisk and pulsatile. Because the flow through a micropuncture needle is six times less, the backflow may not appear pulsatile.

18 gauge needle steps

- The 0.035″ guidewire is threaded through the needle. There should be no resistance as the wire is advanced. If resistance is encountered, fluoroscopy should be employed to ensure proper wire advancement (Fig. 2.2. Step II a, b, and c).
- After the sheath and dilator are advanced over the wire, the dilator and wire are removed (Fig. 2.2. Step II d and e).

Micropuncture steps

- Access the arterial as described above with the needle found in the micropuncture access kit. Once the arterial access is obtained, the accompanying 0.018″ guidewire is advanced through the needle (Fig. 2.2. Step III a). Because the wire is straight (not J-tipped), it is essential to check by fluoroscopy that the wire tip is in the iliac artery and has not advanced into a small branch (Fig. 2.2. Step III b).
- Thread the 2F dilator accompanying the 4F sheath dilator system over the guidewire into the arterial (Fig. 2.2. Step III c) and remove the guidewire. Perform an arteriogram with a 3 cc injection of dye through the 2F dilator to confirm that the site of entry is optimal. If the arterial puncture site is not optimal, remove the catheter, hold pressure for 3–5 min to achieve hemostasis, and access the arterial again with the micropuncture needle.
- Remove the 2F dilator and re-assemble the 4F micropuncture sheath/dilator system and advance the system over the wire (Fig. 2.2. Step III d). Then exchange the 0.018″ wire with a 0.035″ guidewire which is then used to advance the 5 or 6 Fr sheath (Fig. 2.2. Step III e, f, and g).

Angiographic views Once arterial access is obtained, a femoral arteriogram should be obtained by injecting dye through the sheath or micropuncture catheter.

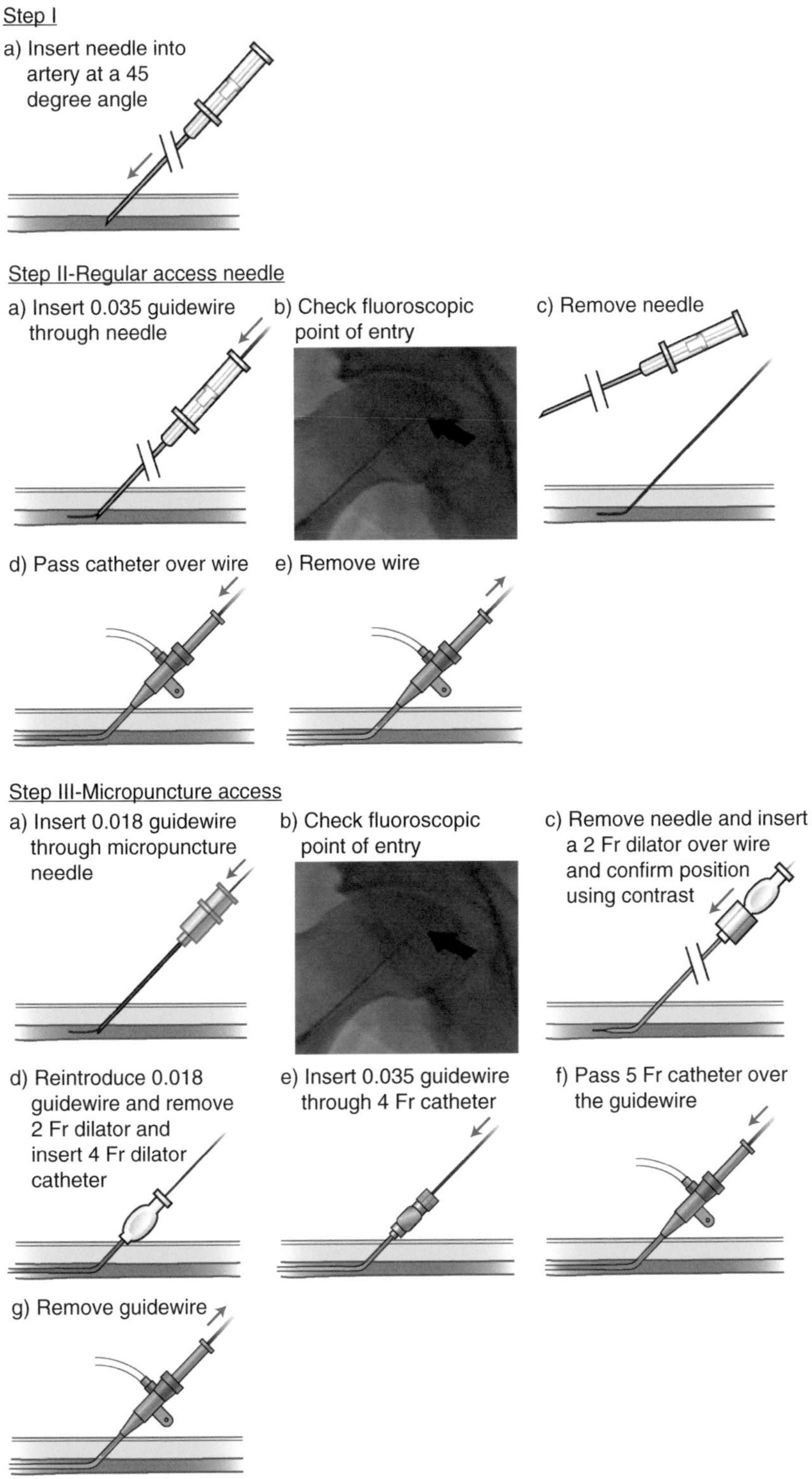

Step I

a) Insert needle into
   artery at a 45
   degree angle

Step II-Regular access needle

a) Insert 0.035 guidewire   b) Check fluoroscopic   c) Remove needle
   through needle   point of entry

d) Pass catheter over wire   e) Remove wire

Step III-Micropuncture access

a) Insert 0.018 guidewire   b) Check fluoroscopic   c) Remove needle and insert
   through micropuncture   point of entry   a 2 Fr dilator over wire
   needle   and confirm position
                                                                       using contrast

d) Reintroduce 0.018   e) Insert 0.035 guidewire   f) Pass 5 Fr catheter over
   guidewire and remove   through 4 Fr catheter   the guidewire
   2 Fr dilator and
   insert 4 Fr dilator
   catheter

g) Remove guidewire

Fig. 2.2 Steps of femoral access

This will allow visualization of the access location in those cases where the micro-puncture access system was not used. The angiogram should be evaluated carefully to see the level of puncture and presence of arterial dissection or extravasation of dye due to peri-sheath leak or back wall puncture.

- Ipsilateral 30 RAO or 30 LAO view for the common femoral artery bifurcation.
- In some cases a contralateral view with a slight caudal projection may allow better visualization of the bifurcation.

Table 2.2 lists the various complications of access sites and their clinical features, prevention, and treatment [2].

Radial Access

Vascular anatomy of the hand

- The ulnar artery and the radial artery provide dual blood supply to the hand and therefore makes partial occlusion of the radial artery during transradial intervention safe (Fig. 2.3).
- The superficial palmar arch lies deep to the palmer fascia and is supplied predominantly by the ulnar artery and to a lesser degree by the superficial branch of the radial artery.
- The deep palmar arch lies deep to the flexor tendons, lies proximal to the superficial arch, and is supplied predominantly by the deep branch of the radial artery and to a lesser degree by the deep branch of the ulnar artery.
- Patients may have variations of this anatomy that limits or precludes dual blood supply to the hand. Therefore it is important to evaluate for the presence of normal anatomy prior to transradial intervention. See section below on Allen's test.

Patient screening and selection Benefits of radial access over femoral access for PCI:

- Clear safety advantage: reduced bleeding and access site complications
- Early ambulation
- Patient comfort and satisfaction

Radial arterial access is a favorable access route for coronary angiography, particularly for those who are high risk for femoral vascular access complications including those with:

- Morbid obesity (>125 kg)
- Severe lower extremity peripheral vascular disease
- Abdominal aortic aneurysm with thrombus
- Anticoagulated patients

Table 2.2 Complications of access sites

Type	Clinical features	Prevention	Treatment
Hematoma	Incidence: 5–23 % Pain, swelling, or hardened area under the skin at site If severe can cause tachycardia, hypotension, and fall in Hct Most resolve in a few weeks	Adequate compression after sheath removal Avoid arterial puncture below the femoral bifurcation	Manual pressure Mark the area to monitor change in size Obtain a vascular ultrasound to evaluate for pseudoaneurysm Other steps same as for retroperitoneal hematoma
Psuedo aneurysm	Incidence: 0.5–9 % Swelling at insertion site Large, painful pulsatile mass Bruit and/or thrill in the groin area Pseudoaneurysm can rupture or cause nerve compression resulting in limb weakness Diagnosed by ultrasound	Adequate compression after sheath removal and good hemostasis Avoid arterial puncture below the femoral bifurcation	Bed rest Small: Monitor as they spontaneously resolve after cessation of anticoagulation Large: manual or ultrasound-guided compression/thrombin injection or surgery
Arteriovenous fistula	Incidence: 0.2–2.1 % Bruit ± thrill at access site Extremity swelling, tenderness Diagnosed by ultrasound	Adequate compression after sheath removal and good hemostasis Avoid arterial puncture below the femoral bifurcation or above inguinal ligament	Some resolve spontaneously Ultrasound-guided compression Surgical repair
Infection [10]	Incidence ~0.4 % 80 % are diabetics with a mortality rate of 6 % 50 % ~ mycotic aneurysm 50 % result in mycotic anuerysm with S. aureus in 75 % of cases S. aureus in 75 % of cases Incubation period is 1 week to 1 month. High degree of suspicion for any pain, erythema, swelling, drainage from the puncture site, or systemic signs of infection up to 1 month post procedure, especially in diabetics	*VCD/manual sheath removal protocol* Clean area with antiseptic solution. Place sterile towels and change gloves. Pull out in one fluid movement and let it bleed back and hold pressure just above puncture site. Do not rub into the wound Avoid VCD in patients with significant PVD, CFA <5 mm, >3 prior procedures at the same site or if puncture is below the femoral bifurcation. Give 1 g of IV Cefazolin or 1 g of IV vancomycin (PCN allergic patients) in DM or morbidly obese patients receiving VCD	Long-term IV antibiotics or antifungals Surgical debridement and removal

Table 2.2 (continued)

Type	Clinical features	Prevention	Treatment
Retro peritoneal hematoma	Incidence: 0.15–0.4 % Moderate to severe abdominal, back, or ipsilateral flank pain Groin/hip pain with radiation to back if close to the iliopsoas muscle especially on extension of the hip Hypotension and tachycardia. Ecchymosis and decrease in hematocrit are late signs Diagnosed by CT Fatal if not recognized early	Avoid puncture above the inguinal ligament Use micropuncture access in obese patients or difficult access and confirm site prior to sheath insertion Adequate compression after sheath removal and good hemostasis	Do not delay treatment if suspicion is high IVF/bed rest Interrupt anticoagulants and antiplatelets with blood transfusion if required May need surgical evacuation/ percutaneous balloon tamponade
Arterial occlusion by thromboembolism (TE)	Incidence: <0.8 % 5 Ps: pain, paralysis, pallor, paresthesias, pulselessness Doppler studies/angiogram	Anticoagulation Vasodilators Careful monitoring during sheath removal and injection	Small TE may undergo spontaneous lysis Larger TE may need surgical or percutaneous thromboembolectomy or thrombolytic agents
	Percutaneous thrombectomy		
	Access from the contralateral side and give 5,000 units of heparin if not anticoagulated		
	Cross TE with a 0.014″ or 0.018″ wire		
	Thrombectomy device is then introduced over the wire to remove any thrombi ± PTA/stent		
Iliac dissection	Usually painless and retrograde		Bed rest with follow-up clinical exams and imaging if nonflow limiting If flow limiting, PTCA + stent is treatment of choice
Femoral neuropathy	Incidence: ~0.2 % Pain ± tingling at access site Numbness ± weakness at access site or down the leg Decreased patellar tendon reflex	Avoid injection or insertion lateral to the arterial pulsation	Physical therapy Local anesthetic injections

Radial artery occlusion	Incidence: 2–18 %	Avoid prolonged periods of high-pressure compression Compression pressure should not occlude flow	Most occlusions are asymptomatic
Radial artery spasm	Incidence: ~2–24 % Challenge for transradial procedures Causing pain and discomfort to the patient	Intra-arterial vasodilator cocktail Hydrophilic sheaths Small-sized sheaths Adequate local anesthesia Adequate patient sedation	Sedation General anesthesia for refractory cases
Radial arterial perforation	Incidence: 0.1–1 % Rare	Avoid aggressive wire manipulation	Pressure bandage for hematoma

Fig. 2.3 Arterial supply of the hand

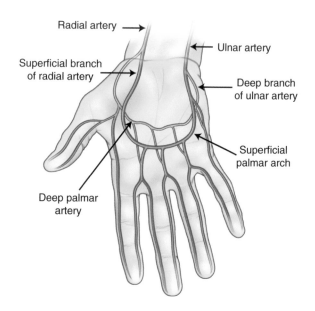

Fig. 2.4 Allen's test, compress the radial and ulnar arteries simultaneously

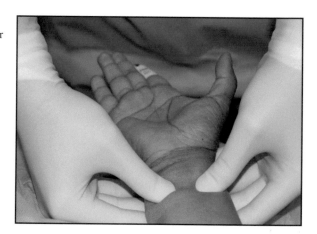

- Patients who cannot lie flat
- Patients with bleeding diathesis

Contraindications for radial access

- Non-palpable radial artery pulse
- Negative Allen's test
- Patient's with existent or AV fistula for dialysis or those at risk for starting dialysis
- INR > 3.5

Fig. 2.5 Release the ulnar artery

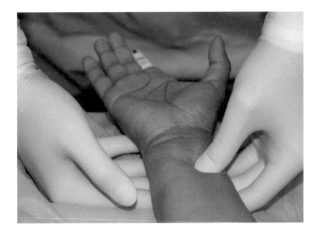

Fig. 2.6 Compress the radial artery and ulnar artery to occlude it for a minute, release the ulnar artery, and observe the pulse wave form of the ulnar artery

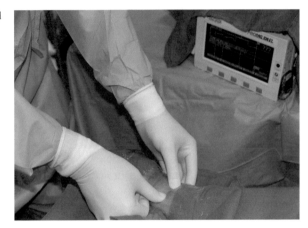

Allen's test

- The patient is first asked to make a fist.
- The operator simultaneously compresses the radial and ulnar arteries with the goal of occluding both arteries (Fig. 2.4).
- The patient is then asked to repeatedly open and close his/her hand five times. The final opened palm should appear blanched.
- Release of the ulnar artery returns the hand color to pink within 8–10 s. A "positive" Allen's test suggests that the ulnar blood supply to the hand will be sufficient if the radial artery is occluded (Fig. 2.5).
- Release of the ulnar artery does not result in return of pink hand color within 8–10 s. A "negative" Allen's test suggests that the ulnar blood supply to the hand will not be sufficient if the radial artery is occluded. Transradial intervention should not be performed.

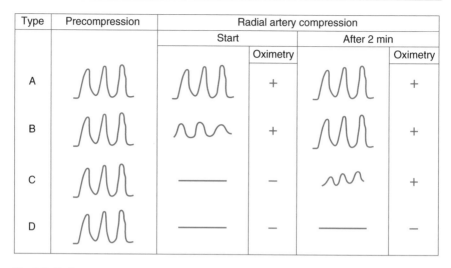

Type	Precompression	Radial artery compression			
		Start	Oximetry	After 2 min	Oximetry
A			+		+
B			+		+
C			–		+
D			–		–

Fig. 2.7 Barbeau test

Allen's oximetry test

- After attaching pulse oximeter to access site hand, observe the pulse wave form.
- Compress the radial artery and ulnar artery to occlude it for a minute, release the ulnar artery, and observe the pulse wave form of the ulnar artery (Fig. 2.6).
- Classify wave form by the Barbeau classification (Fig. 2.7):
  - Type A: no change in pulse wave
  - Type B: a damped but distinct pulse wave form.
  - Type C: a loss of phasic pulse wave form, followed by recovery in 2 minutes
  - Type D: no recovery of pulse tracing within 2 min.
- Radial artery cannulation is not performed for type D wave forms.

Prepping the arm

- The arm is immobilized on the radial arm board.
- The radial wrist is hyperextended with a wrist brace or towelettes.
- A pulse oximeter is placed on the index finger for monitoring during the procedure.

Radial artery puncture and sheath insertion Utilize a Terumo® (Tokyo, Japan) Glidesheath™ radial arterial puncture kit.

- The radial kit contains a 20 gauge SURFLO IV™ catheter, soft mini guidewire, and Glidesheath™ (4 Fr, 5 Fr, 6 Fr). The 6 Fr is generally used so that if intervention is performed, no sheath exchange is necessary.
- Place the hand positioned along the body with the palm pointing upward and obliquely. The use of an arm board with a towel that hyperextends the wrist will

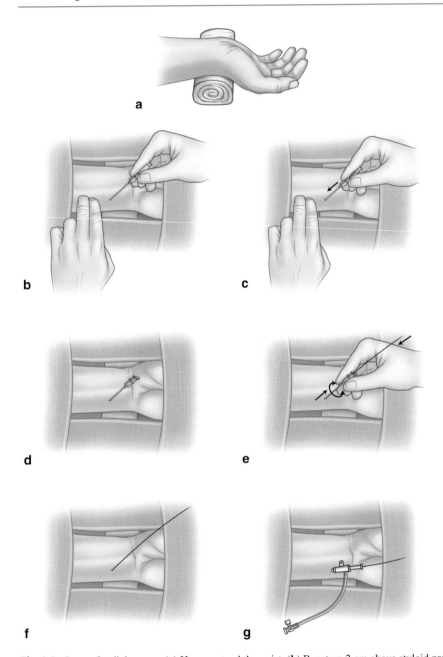

Fig. 2.8 Steps of radial access. (**a**) Hyper-extend the wrist. (**b**) Puncture 2 cm above styloid process. (**c**) Pulsatile blood flow is seen. (**d**) Advance needle more few millimeters. (**e**) Thread the 0.018" guidewire through the needle. (**f**) Remove the needle. (**g**) Insert the Terumo sheath.

make the access easier (Fig. 2.8a). Apply local skin anesthesia with 0.5 ml 1 % lidocaine.

- Radial artery puncture site should be 2 cm proximal to the styloid process (Fig. 2.8b). Utilize the Seldinger technique with back wall puncture. When blood appears in the hub of the IV catheter (Fig. 2.8c), the cannula is advanced a few millimeters through the back wall of the arterial in order to transfix the arterial and subsequently the needle is withdrawn (Fig. 2.8d). The cannula is gently drawn back until pulsatile backflow appears. After gaining pulsatile blood flow, advance soft mini 0.018″ guidewire (Fig. 2.8e) and remove IV catheter (Fig. 2.8f)
- Advance the 10 cm hydrophilic sheath over the mini guidewire (Fig. 2.8g). Typically one can utilize a 6 Fr Terumo® Glidesheath (hydrophilic tapered sheath). Sometimes a 4 or 5 Fr sheath is needed for smaller radial arteries.
- After insertion of a sheath, a cocktail of verapamil (2.5 mg), NTG (~200 mcg, blood pressure permitting), and 2,000–4,000 IU of heparin is prepared in a single 50 cc syringe. Aspirate about 30 cc of blood to dilute the mixture prior to injection to reduce patient discomfort.
- The same steps are used if the operator uses a 21 gauge micropuncture needle instead of the IV catheter. However, an anterior wall puncture is recommended. A through and through puncture of the back wall can induce spasm.
- The same steps are used for left radial access. However, once the sheath is successfully placed, the left arm is draped over the abdomen of the patient so that the operator can stand on the patient's right side.

Pearls

When an IV catheter (such as the one included in the Terumo® kit) is used to obtain access, a back wall puncture is essential. If a micropuncture needle is used, avoid puncturing through the back wall.

When using the IV catheter, ascertaining pulsatile flow is essential before proceeding. Pulsatile flow may not be seen when using a micropuncture needle.

A higher dose of heparin (4,000 IU vs. 2,000 IU) is helpful in preventing radial artery occlusion.

Avoiding radial artery spasm

- Predictors of spasm:
  - Young patients
  - Women
  - Low BMI
  - Small radial artery diameter
  - Large sheath size
  - Multiple access attempts
  - Number of catheter and procedure duration

- Prevention:
  - Proper sedation
  - Local anesthesia
  - NTG (~200 mcg, depending on BP)
  - Verapamil (2.5 mg)
  - Smooth wiring of the vessel without undue force and gentle sheath insertion employing hydrophilic sheaths with tapered dilators

Pearl
The comfortably sedated patient in no pain will be less likely to have radial artery spasm.

References

1. Dehmer GJ, Weaver D, Roe MT, Milford-Beland S, Fitzgerald S, Hermann A, Messenger J, Moussa I, Garratt K, Rumsfeld J, Brindis RG. A contemporary view of diagnostic cardiac catheterization and percutaneous coronary intervention in the United States: a report from the CathPCI Registry of the National Cardiovascular Data Registry, 2010 through June 2011. J Am Coll Cardiol. 2012;60:2017–31. PMID: 23083784.
2. Sherev DA, Shaw RE, Brent BN. Angiographic predictors of femoral access site complications: implication for planned percutaneous coronary intervention. Catheter Cardiovasc Interv. 2005;65:196–202. PMID: 15895402.
3. Kiviniemi T, Karjalainen P, Pietilä M, Ylitalo A, Niemelä M, Vikman S, Puurunen M, Biancari F, Airaksinen KE. Comparison of additional versus no additional heparin during therapeutic oral anticoagulation in patients undergoing percutaneous coronary intervention. Am J Cardiol. 2012;110:30–5. PMID: 22464216.
4. Fenger-Eriksen C, Münster AM, Grove EL. New oral anticoagulants: clinical indications, monitoring and treatment of acute bleeding complications. Acta Anaesthesiol Scand. 2014;58:651–9. PMID: 24716468.
5. Ahmed B, Lischke S, Holterman LA, Straight F, Dauerman HL. Angiographic predictors of vascular complications among women undergoing cardiac catheterization and intervention. J Invasive Cardiol. 2010;22:512–6. PMID: 21041845.
6. Garrett PD, Eckart RE, Bauch TD, Thompson CM, Stajduhar KC. Fluoroscopic localization of the femoral head as a landmark for common femoral artery cannulation. Catheter Cardiovasc Interv. 2005;65:205–7. PMID:15900552.
7. Spijkerboer AM, Scholten FG, Mali WP, van Schaik JP. Antegrade puncture of the femoral artery: morphologic study. Radiology. 1990;176:57–60. PMID:2353111.
8. Grier D, Hartnell G. Percutaneous femoral artery puncture: practice and anatomy. Br J Radiol. 1990;63:602–4. PMID: 2400874 (femoral pulse).
9. Lechner G, Jantsch H, Waneck R, Kretschmer G. The relationship between the common femoral artery, the inguinal crease, and the inguinal ligament: a guide to accurate angiographic puncture. Cardiovasc Intervent Radiol. 1988;11:165–9. PMID: 3139299.
10. Sohail MR, Khan AH, Holmes Jr DR, Wilson WR, Steckelberg JM, Baddour LM. Infectious complications of percutaneous vascular closure devices. Mayo Clin Proc. 2005;80:1011–5. PMID: 16092579.

The Perfect Shot: Angiographic Views for the Interventionalist

3

Anitha Rajamanickam and Annapoorna Kini

Introduction

The most important function of coronary angiography is to accurately define coronary anatomy and obtain optimal and comprehensive angiographic views of the entire course of the main epicardial coronary arteries and their branches to aid in the diagnosis of and the therapeutic interventions for coronary artery disease. The key is to maintain a fine balance between harmful radiation and dye exposure and essential number of images obtained to clearly define the anatomy. Inadequate knowledge of the best views and suboptimal angiographic images can lead to serious consequences of either missing disease or inappropriate interventions and wasteful healthcare expenditure.

Our Protocol

In most cases, for a right dominant system, we have found that the left coronary system can be adequately visualized in three views and the right system in one to two views. The views are named in the following order:

- The first number denotes left anterior oblique (LAO) and right anterior oblique (RAO) angles or anteroposterior(AP) view.
- The second number denotes straight or cranial/caudal angulation.

A. Rajamanickam, MD (✉) • A. Kini, MD, MRCP, FACC
Department of Interventional Cardiology, Mount Sinai Hospital,
One Gustave Levy Place, Madison Avenue, New York, NY 10029, USA
e-mail: arajamanickam@gmail.com, Anitha.Rajamanickam@mountsinai.org;
Annapoorna.kini@mountsinai.org

© Springer-Verlag London 2014
A. Kini et al. (eds.), *Practical Manual of Interventional Cardiology*,
DOI 10.1007/978-1-4471-6581-1_3

23

Left System

- *LAO caudal/spider view* [40, 40]: The left main trunk (LMT) and its bifurcation into the proximal left anterior descending (LAD) artery and proximal left circumflex (LCX) artery or trifurcation if the ramus intermedius (RI) is present
- *RAO caudal* [20, 20]: LMT, proximal LAD, LCX, and obtuse marginal (OM) branches
- *RAO Cranial* [10, 40]: Mid and distal LAD and separation of septal and diagonal branches
- *LAO cranial* [30, 30]: If it is left dominant system to visualize, the left posterior descending artery (LPDA)

The Right Coronary Artery

- *LAO cranial* [30, 30]: Visualize the right posterior descending artery (RPDA), AV continuation, and right posterolateral (RPL) bifurcation
- *LAO* [30, 0]: Proximal, mid, and distal right coronary artery (RCA)

To Define Specific Lesions

We use the following views for better definition of specific lesions:

- *LM*:
    - Ostial: RAO cranial, AP cranial, LAO cranial
    - Body: RAO caudal, AP caudal, LAO caudal
- *LAD*:
    - Ostial/proximal: spider, LAO cranial
    - Mid/distal: AP cranial, RAO cranial
- *Diagonal*:
    - Origin: LAO cranial, LAO caudal
    - Mid/distal: AP cranial, RAO cranial
- *Septals*: RAO cranial, AP cranial
- *Ramus*:
    - Ostial/proximal: spider, AP caudal
    - Distal: AP caudal
- *Circumflex*:
    - Ostial/proximal: spider, AP caudal
    - Mid/distal: AP cranial, RAO cranial
- *OM*:
    - Ostial/proximal: RAO caudal.
    - Mid/distal: AP cranial, RAO cranial.

- LPDA: LAO cranial, AP cranial. In a left dominant system, the LPDA and posterior left ventricle branches are seen clearly because they circle beneath the LAD.
- *RCA*
  - Ostial/proximal: LAO caudal
  - Mid: RAO 30°
  - Distal: AP cranial/RAO cranial/LAO cranial
  - PDA/RPL: AP cranial/RAO cranial
  - Early bifurcating RPDA: RAO 30°

Grafts

- *LIMA:*
  - Ostium/body: AP straight [0, 0]
  - Anastomosis to LAD: RAO 30° AP cranial
  - LAD after anastomosis: AP cranial
- *RIMA:*
  - Ostium/body: AP straight [0, 0]
  - Anastomosis and vessel after anastomosis: will depend on vessel bypassed
- *SVG:*
  - Ostium/body: LAO 30°, RAO 30°
  - Anastomosis to RCA/PDA/PL: RAO cranial
  - Anastomosis to LCX/OM/Ramus: RAO caudal
  - Anastomosis to LAD/Diagonol: AP cranial
  - Native vessel after anastomosis: depends on vessel involved (see above)

Collaterals

- Left to right: LAO cranial
- Right to left: RAO straight

Physiological Assessment During Interventional Procedures

4

Nagendra Boopathy Senguttuvan, Anitha Rajamanickam, and Annapoorna Kini

Angiography identifies the minimal luminal diameter but does not calculate the minimal luminal area. The operator should keep in mind the limitations of angiography. A significant lesion may be missed due to its eccentric nature, ostial position or location in a highly tortuous artery. In addition, moderate (50–70 %) lesions may be hemodynamically significant (see Fig. 4.1). Fractional flow reserve [FFR] provides objective evidence for functional significance. FFR-guided decision making provides better clinical outcomes when compared to angiography, and therefore every operator must be well versed this technique [1].

Definition

FFR is the ratio of pressures distal [Pd] to and proximal [Pa] to the stenotic lesions at hyperemic flow. It relates epicardial stenosis to myocardial blood flow and area.

Characteristics

- Independent of HR/BP/LV function
- Accounts for collaterals
- Easy to perform and interpret
- Reproducible
- Directly relates the myocardial blood flow
- Excellent correlation with noninvasive tests

N.B. Senguttuvan, MD, DM (✉) • A. Rajamanickam, MD • A. Kini, MD, MRCP, FACC (✉)
Department of Interventional Cardiology, Mount Sinai Hospital,
One Gustave Levy Place, Madison Avenue, New York, NY 10029, USA
e-mail: drsnboopathy@gmail.com; arajamanickam@gmail.com; anitha.rajamanickam@mountsinai.org; Annapoorna.kini@mountsinai.org

© Springer-Verlag London 2014
A. Kini et al. (eds.), *Practical Manual of Interventional Cardiology*,
DOI 10.1007/978-1-4471-6581-1_4

Fig. 4.1 LAO caudal view
showing angiographically
significant ostial OM1
stenosis which was FFR
negative. *Arrow* denotes FFR
of the indicated lesions

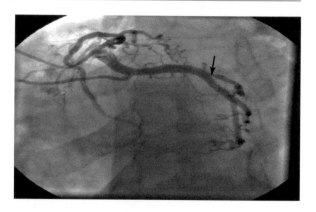

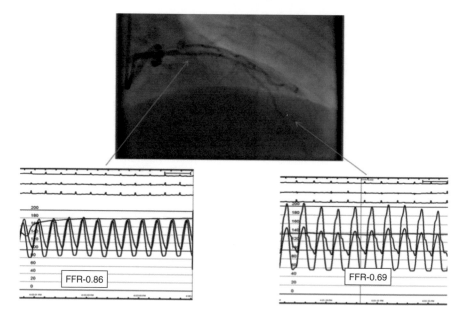

Fig. 4.2 Hemodynamic assessment of proximal and distal LAD lesion by FFR

Value of FFR

In a vessel without any obstructions, the value of FFR is 1. Based on FAME and
FAME II trials [1, 2], FFR ≤0.8 is considered significant and may benefit from
CI (see Fig. 4.2). Patient with FFR >0.8 has excellent prognosis with medical
therapy alone. Only 0.2 % of FFR-negative patients had an MI at 2 years
follow-up.

Drugs Used

Adenosine

IV: Preferred over a central line or a large bore peripheral line 140 mcg/kg/min infusion

IC: LCA, 80–120 mcg bolus. Bolus repeated three times. Lower dose 60–80 mcg bolus for RCA

Role of FFR

- Multivessel disease
- Left main disease
- Ostial lesion
- Multiple lesions in a single vessel
- Bifurcation

Steps of FFR

- Anticoagulation as per institution protocol.
- Flush the pressure wire system with saline and keep it flat on the table.
- Zero the pressure wire system and remove the FFR wire carefully.
- Pressure sensor is located at the junction between the radiolucent and the radiopaque portion of the wire.
- Advance the wire into the proximal part of the vessel so that the pressure sensor is proximal to the stenosis and remove the introducer needle. Flush the guide catheter system with saline while holding the wire and then equalize. The difference between Pa and Pd pressure tracings [Offset] after equalizing to "1.00" should not be greater than 15. If the Offset is greater than 15 the FFR readings are not valid.
- For LM/ostial main vessel stenosis, always disengage the guide and equalize in the aorta.
- Once equalized, reintroduce the wire introducer and advance the FFR wire distal to the lesion. Start vasodilators as per protocol.
- While removing the wire, reconfirm that both the pressures are equal once the radiopaque part of the wire is pulled back proximal to the lesion.
- Take a final angiogram to ensure that there were no complications from the FFR wire.

FFR of Multiple Lesions in Same Vessel

- Consider the FFR as the FFR of the entire vessel rather than that of individual lesions.
- If FFR >0.8, none of the lesions are significant. No intervention is required.
- For tandem and sequential lesions, the maximum drop in mean pressure should be observed. In Fig. 4.3, FFR of the vessel with two tandem lesions is ≤0.8 and

Proximal   Distal

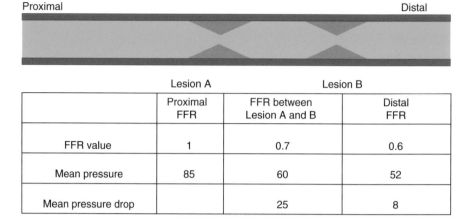

| | Lesion A | | Lesion B |
	Proximal FFR	FFR between Lesion A and B	Distal FFR
FFR value	1	0.7	0.6
Mean pressure	85	60	52
Mean pressure drop		25	8

Fig. 4.3 Clinical example showing two lesions and FFR readings

Proximal   Distal

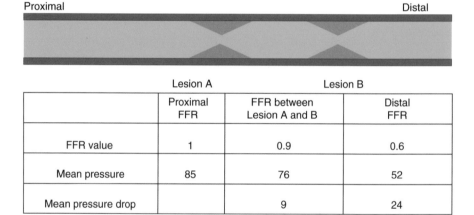

| | Lesion A | | Lesion B |
	Proximal FFR	FFR between Lesion A and B	Distal FFR
FFR value	1	0.9	0.6
Mean pressure	85	76	52
Mean pressure drop		9	24

Fig. 4.4 Clinical example showing two lesions and FFR readings

the drop in mean pressure is more for the proximal lesion than the distal lesion. Here the proximal lesion needs to be treated first. In Fig. 4.4, FFR of the vessel with two tandem lesions is ≤0.8 but the drop in mean pressure is more for the distal lesion than the proximal lesion. Here the distal lesion needs to be treated first. After the first intervention, the second lesion may be reassessed. This is true for all lesions in series in a vessel except for left main disease. If the two lesions are close enough, a single stent covering both lesions may be considered.

Left Main Disease FFR

FFR values (>0.80) in left main lesions are associated with excellent long-term outcomes. Presence of downstream disease may affect the FFR value of LM disease. Myocardial bed supplied by the LM artery may be larger if it supplies collaterals to an occluded RCA. It is postulated that the presence of significant lesion in either the LAD or the LCX makes the myocardial bed smaller for the LM leading to a falsely higher FFR. The left main FFR alone cannot be accurately measured when there are significant downstream serial lesions. If the LAD and LCX are hemodynamically insignificant, the left main FFR will be accurate. Use smaller (6 Fr), less aggressive guides (FL,VL) for the procedure in order to avoid LM dissection at the site of lesion.

SVG Lesion

The role of FFR in SVG lesion is controversial as the distal coronary pressure represents blood flow due to both SVG and a non-occluded native vessel.

Acute MI

The role of FFR in STEMI is controversial due to microvascular obstruction from thrombus embolization and vasospasm associated with infarct. After an MI, the FFR may be normal even though angiographically the obstruction is significant. This may be due to the fact that the infarcted territory has more of scar tissue and less of viable tissue rather than a false underestimation of FFR provided maximal hyperemia is obtained.

In-Stent Restenosis

The role of FFR has not been well defined in ISR and the lesion should be assessed by IVUS if needed.

Troubleshooting

Improper preparation/setup

- Height of the fluid-filled pressure transducer. An increase or decrease in 10 cm from the mid atrial level leads to change in aortic pressure by 10 mmHg.
- Make sure you have flushed the system with normal saline before zeroing the FFR wire.
- Equalize the pressure wire with guide catheter pressure appropriately.
- Flush the system with normal saline before equalizing as presence of contrast will lead to pressure damping.
- Remove the introducer needle from the Y connector before equalizing the pressures.

Inadequate hyperemia Obtaining hyperemia is the single most important step in assessing lesion significance by FFR. Submaximal hyperemia is indicated by an undulating FFR Pd/Pa tracing. Increasing dose of adenosine has been shown to produce maximal hyperemia.

Pressure drift Presence of FFR ≤0.8 with same pressure trace in the aorta and distal coronary artery is likely due to pressure drift. Absence of ventricularized pattern of distal pressure trace rules out an abnormal FFR due to an epicardial vessel stenosis.

Guide catheter issues

- Larger guide catheter leads to lumen narrowing leading to falsely higher FFR.
- Diagnostic catheter with narrow lumen leads to aortic pressure dampening leading to falsely higher FFR.
- Avoid using side-hole catheters.
- For LM/ostial stenosis always disengage the guide and equalize with wire in the aorta.

Whipping artifacts If the coronary wire touches the wall, whipping artifact occurs leading to falsely high coronary pressure. This can be managed by pulling the wire or advancing it 2–3 mm.

Difficulty in crossing the lesion Use another wire as a buddy wire to cross the lesion with FFR wire.

References

1. Tonino PA, De Bruyne B, Pijls NH. Fractional flow reserve versus angiography for guiding percutaneous coronary intervention. N Engl J Med. 2009;360(3):213–24
2. De Bruyne B, Pijls NH, Kalesan B. Fractional flow reserve-guided PCI versus medical therapy in stable coronary disease. N Engl J Med. 2012;367(11):991–1001.

Antiplatelet and Antithrombotic Therapy in PCI

5

Rikesh Patel, Anitha Rajamanickam, and Annapoorna Kini

Advances in drug stent-eluting technology, antiplatelet pharmacotherapy, and novel parenteral and oral anticoagulants have led to a constant evolution in periprocedural antithrombotic strategy. The following chapter outlines our cardiac catheterization laboratory's current approach to antiplatelet and anticoagulation therapy in various clinical settings based on current guidelines, data, and expert opinion.

Oral Antiplatelet Therapy

Aspirin – all patients

- For elective patients, with or without known stable CAD, aspirin 162 mg should be given at time of obtaining consent.
- For ACS (acute coronary syndrome) patients, non-enteric aspirin 325 mg should be given as early as possible prior to PCI.
- Post-PCI, aspirin 81 mg daily should be continued indefinitely.

Dual antiplatelet therapy

- All patients should be counseled on the necessity of and concomitant risk associated with dual antiplatelet therapy (DAPT) prior to placement of intracoronary stents, especially drug-eluting stents (DES).

R. Patel, MD • A. Rajamanickam, MD • A. Kini, MD, MRCP, FACC (✉)
Department of Interventional Cardiology, Mount Sinai Hospital,
One Gustave Levy Place, Madison Avenue, New York, NY 10029, USA
e-mail: rikeshrpatel@gmail.com, rikeshpatel.md@gmail.com; arajamanickam@gmail.com,
anitha.rajamanickam@mountsinai.org; Annapoorna.kini@mountsinai.org

© Springer-Verlag London 2014
A. Kini et al. (eds.), *Practical Manual of Interventional Cardiology*,
DOI 10.1007/978-1-4471-6581-1_5

- For patients unable or unwilling to comply with recommended duration of dual antiplatelet therapy, alternative revascularization (bypass) or bare metal stents (BMS) should be considered.

P2Y12 antagonist therapy

- Pre-/intra-procedural loading doses for patients *not previously taking the same* P2Y12 receptor inhibitor for ≥5 days:
  - Clopidogrel 600 mg (patients who received fibrinolytics <24 h should receive a 300 mg loading dose if they are <75 years of age and 75 mg loading dose if >75 years of age)
  - Prasugrel 60 mg
  - Ticagrelor 180 mg
- Loading doses for patients *already taking the same* P2Y12 receptor inhibitor for ≥5 days:
  - Clopidogrel 300 mg
  - Prasugrel 30 mg
  - Ticagrelor 90 mg
- For clopidogrel *nonresponders* (with confirmed compliance), defined as platelet reactivity unit (PRU) >230, load with prasugrel 60 mg or ticagrelor 180 mg.

Special considerations

- In patients who received fibrinolytics <24 h, only clopidogrel should be used.
- Prasugrel (contraindicated in patients with a history of TIA/CVA and avoided in patients weighing >60 kg or >75 years of age) should be preferred in the following clinical situations:
  - STEMI
  - Diabetics with multivessel disease
  - Clopidogrel allergy
  - Clopidogrel nonresponder (PRU >230 on maintenance dose of clopidogrel)
  - Stent thrombosis on clopidogrel
- In patients *>75 years old or with history of TIA/CVA, or weighing <60 kg,* ticagrelor should be preferred in the following clinical situations:
  - NSTEMI
  - Complex PCI
  - Clopidogrel allergy
  - Clopidogrel nonresponder (PRU >230 on maintenance dose of clopidogrel)
  - Stent thrombosis on clopidogrel
- For *pre-liver* transplant patients, BMS are preferred to enable shorter duration of DAPT, with the exception of left main, bifurcation, or proximal LAD lesions, where DES may be preferred.
- For *pre-renal* transplant patients, DES are generally preferred, unless a transplant date is set within 1–4 months.

Table 5.1 Duration of DAPT

Duration of pharmacotherapy				
		Antiplatelet		Anticoagulant
		Aspirin 81 mg	P2Y12 antagonist	Warfarin[a]
Bleed risk	Stent type	Daily	Prasugrel Ticagrelor Clopidogrel	Dabigatran[b] Apixaban[b] Rivaroxaban[b]
Low	DES	3 months	Indefinitely	Indefinitely
Low	BMS	1 month	Indefinitely	Indefinitely
High	DES	1 month	Indefinitely	Indefinitely
High	BMS	1 month	Indefinitely	Indefinitely

[a]*Non-valvular* AF, the goal INR 2–2.5; *valvular* AF, mechanical valve, thromboembolism: goal INR 2.5–3
[b]Only approved for *non-valvular* AF; dosing should be adjusted for renal impairment, weight, drug interactions

Duration of DAPT (See Table 5.1)

- All ACS patients should receive 12 months of DAPT.
- Non-ACS patients receiving DES should receive 12 months of DAPT.
- Non-ACS patients receiving BMS should receive 1 month of DAPT.
- Prolonged DAPT beyond 12 months may be considered in patients tolerating therapy without bleeding issues, with complex disease requiring multiple stents, and/or significant residual CAD.
- Combined dosing for P2Y12 antagonists with aspirin 81 mg daily:
  - Clopidogrel 75 mg orally once daily
  - Prasugrel 5 mg orally once daily (10 mg daily in patients >100 kg)
  - Ticagrelor 90 mg orally twice daily

Antiplatelet therapy in PCI patients requiring oral anticoagulation

- All patients are loaded with aspirin and P2Y12 antagonist, regardless of long-term anticoagulant requirement.
- Patients at *high*-risk for bleeding:
  - History of prior bleeding
  - Age >75 years
  - Renal insufficiency (chronic kidney disease stage 3, estimated glomerular filtration rate <60 mL/min/1.73 m^2)
  - Uncontrolled hypertension
  - History of peptic ulcer disease
  - Baseline anemia, thrombocytopenia (hematocrit <28 %, platelets <100 K)
- In patients at higher risk for bleeding, clopidogrel is preferred as the initial P2Y12 antagonist of choice. If the patient is a clopidogrel nonresponder, ticagrelor is the next preferred option. Prasugrel is generally avoided for patients on warfarin [1].

- For duration of antiplatelet therapy in the setting of long-term anticoagulation, see Table 5.1.
- Post-PCI resumption of anticoagulant therapy [2–6]:
  - Warfarin should be dosed the *same day/evening* due to expected delay in achieving therapeutic INR range.
  - New oral anticoagulants should be dosed the *following day*, unless there is a compelling indication for immediate resumption (below) [7].
  - In patients with compelling indications requiring immediate anticoagulation (or re-bridge to oral anticoagulation) post PCI, such as acute venous/pulmonary thromboembolism or mechanical valve, a heparin drip may be started without bolus 2 h post PCI with successful hemostasis using a closure device or 6 h after sheath pull with successful hemostasis using manual compression.

Anticoagulation for PCI

- Administer bivalirudin bolus (0.75 mg/kg) via the intra-arterial sheath and begin continuous infusion (1.75 mg/kg/h).
- Check activated clotting time (ACT) 3 min after bolus:
  - For ACT <250, administer additional 1/2 bolus of bivalirudin.
  - For ACT 251–299, administer additional 1/3 bolus of bivalirudin.
  - Guiding catheter may be inserted once ACT> 200.
  - Intracoronary guidewire/equipment may be inserted once ACT >300.
- Post PCI:
  - For patients naïve to clopidogrel (on therapy <1 week or receiving the first time load of 600 mg <2 h prior to PCI), bivalirudin infusion should be continued for 2 h from time of stent implantation.
  - For patients receiving prasugrel or ticagrelor (on maintenance therapy or receiving the first time load on the table), bivalirudin infusion can be discontinued as soon as the PCI is completed.
  - For patients requiring an periprocedural glycoprotein (GP) IIb/IIIa inhibitor bolus, bivalirudin infusion can be stopped after administration of the GP IIb/IIIa bolus.

Parenteral antiplatelet therapy

- Due to up-front loading of P2Y12 antagonists and standard use of bivalirudin for anticoagulation during PCI, in our practice, we reserve GP IIb/IIIa antagonist administration for bailout purposes only.
- At the discretion of the operator, single (or double) bolus eptifibatide (single = 180 mcg/kg) may be administered in cases of *edge dissection, side branch closure, slow flow, no reflow, embolization,* and *thrombus* [8].
- For patients receiving abciximab, platelet count should be checked 3 h post procedure and the following morning.
- For patients receiving eptifibatide, platelet count should be checked 6 h post procedure and the following morning.

- In the rare case that GPIIb/IIIa infusion is utilized, the infusion should be discontinued if any significant thrombocytopenia develops (platelets <100 K).
- Protocol for post-procedural thrombocytopenia.

Platelets <20 K

- Discontinue all antiplatelet therapies.
- Transfuse 5 or more units of platelets until platelet count >20 K.
- Aspirin 81 mg and clopidogrel 75 mg can be resumed once platelet count >50 K.
- Platelet count should be checked daily until >70 K.

Platelets 20–50 K

- Discontinue GP2b3a inhibitor.
- Transfuse platelets only for active bleeding.
- Aspirin 81 mg and clopidogrel 75 mg can be resumed once platelet count >50 K.

Platelets 50–100 K

- Discontinue GP2b3a inhibitor.
- Aspirin 81 mg and clopidogrel 75 mg can be continued as long as platelet count remains >50 K.

References

1. Gallagher AM, van Staa TP, Murray-Thomas T, et al. Population-based cohort study of warfarin-treated patients with atrial fibrillation: incidence of cardiovascular and bleeding outcomes. BMJ Open. 2014;4:e003839.
2. Go AS, Hylek EM, Chang Y, et al. Anticoagulation therapy for stroke prevention in atrial fibrillation: how well do randomized trials translate into clinical practice? JAMA. 2003;290:268.
3. Gage BF, Waterman AD, Shannon W, et al. Validation of clinical classification schemes for predicting stroke: results from the National Registry of Atrial Fibrillation. JAMA. 2001;285:2864.
4. Lip GY. Implications of the CHA2DS2-VASc and HAS-BLED Scores for thromboprophylaxis in atrial fibrillation. Am J Med. 2011;124:111.
5. Dewilde WJ, Oirbans T, Verheugt FW, et al. Use of clopidogrel with or without aspirin in patients taking oral anticoagulant therapy and undergoing percutaneous coronary intervention: an open-label, randomised, controlled trial. Lancet. 2013;381:1107.
6. National Collaborating Centre for Chronic Conditions. Atrial fibrillation: national clinical guideline for management in primary and secondary care. London: Royal College of Physicians; 2006.
7. European Heart Rhythm Association, European Association for Cardio-Thoracic Surgery, Camm AJ, et al. Guidelines for the management of atrial fibrillation: the Task Force for the Management of Atrial Fibrillation of the European Society of Cardiology (ESC). Eur Heart J. 2010;31:2369.
8. O'shea JC, Madan M, Cantor WJ, et al. Design and methodology of the ESPRIT trial: evaluating a novel dosing regimen of eptifibatide in percutaneous coronary intervention. Am Heart J. 2000;149(2):S36–43.

Patient Selection and Appropriateness

6

Anitha Rajamanickam and Samin Sharma

The American College of Cardiology Foundation (ACCF), American Heart Association (AHA), Society for Cardiovascular Angiography and Interventions (SCAI), Society of Thoracic Surgeons (STS), and American Association for Thoracic Surgery (AATS) published appropriate use criteria (AUC) for coronary revascularization (Fig. 6.1) to guide physicians to delivering high-quality care to patients with cardiovascular diseases. These guidelines are either evidence based or are expert consensus opinion (when evidence is lacking) and are approved by ACCF and the AHA.

Appropriate Use Criteria (AUC)

AUC are based on the following three criteria:

- Risk level of noninvasive stress tests (see Table 6.1)
- Anti-ischemic medical therapy: patients are considered to be on maximal anti-ischemic medical therapy (MMT) if they are compliant with maximally tolerated prescribed doses of at least 2 of the following classes of drugs to reduce anginal symptoms (beta-blockers, calcium channel blockers, long-acting nitrates, ranolazine)
- Symptoms (see Table 6.2)

A. Rajamanickam, MD (✉) • S. Sharma, MD, FACC
Department of Interventional Cardiology, Mount Sinai Hospital,
One Gustave Levy Place, Madison Avenue, New York, NY 10029, USA
e-mail: arajamanickam@gmail.com, Anitha.Rajamanickam@mountsinai.org;
Samin.sharma@mountsinai.org

© Springer-Verlag London 2014
A. Kini et al. (eds.), *Practical Manual of Interventional Cardiology*,
DOI 10.1007/978-1-4471-6581-1_6

Low-Risk Findings on Noninvasive Study

Symptoms Med. Rx	CTO of 1-vz.; no other disease	1-2-vz. disease; no prox. LAD	1-vz. disease of prox. LAD	2-vz. disease with prox. LAD	3-vz. disease; no left main
Class III or IV Max Rx	U	A	A	A	A
Class I or II Max Rx	U	U	A	A	A
Asymptomatic Max Rx	I	I	U	U	U
Class III or IV No/min Rx	I	U	A	A	A
Class I or II No/min Rx	I	I	U	U	U
Asymptomatic No/min Rx	I	I	U	U	U

Asymptomatic

Stress Test Med. Rx	CTO of 1-vz.; no other disease	1-2-vz. disease; no prox. LAD	1-vz. disease of prox. LAD	2-vz. disease with prox. LAD	3-vz. disease; no left main
High Risk Max Rx	U	A	A	A	A
High Risk No/min Rx	U	U	A	A	A
Int. Risk Max Rx	U	U	U	U	A
Int. Risk No/min Rx	I	I	U	U	A
Low Risk Max Rx	I	I	U	U	U
Low Risk No/min Rx	I	I	U	U	U

Intermediate Risk Findings on Noninvasive Study

Symptoms Med. Rx	CTO of 1-vz.; no other disease	1-2-vz. disease; no prox. LAD	1-vz. disease of prox. LAD	2-vz. disease with prox. LAD	3-vz. disease; no left main
Class III or IV Max Rx	A	A	A	A	A
Class I or II Max Rx	U	A	A	A	A
Asymptomatic Max Rx	U	U	U	U	A
Class III or IV No/min Rx	U	U	A	A	A
Class I or II No/min Rx	U	U	U	A	A
Asymptomatic No/min Rx	I	I	U	U	A

CCS Class I or II Angina

Stress Test Med. Rx	CTO of 1-vz.; no other disease	1-2-vz. disease; no prox. LAD	1-vz. disease of prox. LAD	2-vz. disease with prox. LAD	3-vz. disease; no left main
High Risk Max Rx	A	A	A	A	A
High Risk No/min Rx	U	A	A	A	A
Int. Risk Max Rx	U	A	A	A	A
Int. Risk No/min Rx	U	U	U	A	A
Low Risk Max Rx	U	U	A	A	A
Low Risk No/min Rx	I	I	U	U	U

High-Risk Findings on Noninvasive Study

Symptoms Med. Rx	CTO of 1-vz.; no other disease	1-2-vz. disease; no prox. LAD	1-vz. disease of prox. LAD	2-vz. disease with prox. LAD	3-vz. disease; no left main
Class III or IV Max Rx	A	A	A	A	A
Class I or II Max Rx	A	A	A	A	A
Asymptomatic Max Rx	U	A	A	A	A
Class III or IV No/min Rx	A	A	A	A	A
Class I or II No/min Rx	U	A	A	A	A
Asymptomatic No/min Rx	U	U	A	A	A

CCS Class III or IV Angina

Stress Test Med. Rx	CTO of 1-vz.; no other disease	1-2-vz. disease; no prox. LAD	1-vz. disease of prox. LAD	2-vz. disease with prox. LAD	3-vz. disease; no left main
High Risk Max Rx	A	A	A	A	A
High Risk No/min Rx	A	A	A	A	A
Int. Risk Max Rx	A	A	A	A	A
Int. Risk No/min Rx	U	U	A	A	A
Low Risk Max Rx	U	A	A	A	A
Low Risk No/min Rx	I	U	A	A	A

	CABG	PCI
Two-vessel CAD with proximal LAD stenosis	A	A
Three-vessel CAD with low CAD burden (i.e., three focal stenosis, low SYNTAX score)	A	A
Three-vessel CAD with intermediate to high CAD burden (i.e., multiple diffuse lesions, presence of CTO, or high SYNTAX score)	A	U
Isolated left main stenosis	A	U
Left main stenosis and additional CAD with low CAD burden (i.e., one to two vessel additional involvement, low SYNTAX score)	A	U
Left main stenosis and additional CAD with intermediate to high CAD burden (i.e., three vessel involvement, presence of CTO, or high SYNTAX score)	A	I

Fig. 6.1 Appropriate use criteria for coronary revascularization (Reprinted from Patel et al. [1] with permission from Elsevier and *Journal of The American College of Cardiology*)

Table 6.1 Risk level of noninvasive stress test findings

1. *Low-risk stress test findings: cardiac mortality of ≤1 % per year*

    (a) *EF*: normal at rest (50 % and above)

    (b) *Treadmill:* low-risk Duke Treadmill Score (+5 and above)

    (c) *Stress nuclear*: normal or small myocardial perfusion defect at rest or with stress

    (d) *Stress echo*: normal or no change of limited resting wall motion abnormalities during stress

    (e) *If a stress test is unavailable, then it is classified as low risk*

2. *Intermediate-risk stress test findings: cardiac mortality of 1–3 % per year*

    (a) *EF*: mild/moderate dysfunction at rest (35–49 %)

    (b) *Treadmill*: intermediate-risk Duke Treadmill Score (from −11 to +4)

    (c) *Stress nuclear*: stress-induced moderate myocardial perfusion defect without increased lung uptake (when using thallium-201) or with LV dilation

    (d) *Stress echo*: wall motion abnormality (no more than 2 segments) only at higher doses of dobutamine

3. *High-risk stress test findings: cardiac mortality of ≥3 % per year*

    (a) *EF*: severe dysfunction at rest or with exercise (<35 %)

    (b) *Treadmill*: high-risk Duke Treadmill Score (less than −11)

    (c) *Stress nuclear*:

    Stress-induced large myocardial perfusion defect

    Stress-induced multiple moderate-sized defects

    Stress-induced moderate-sized defect with either increased lung uptake (thallium-201) or LV dilation

    Large, fixed perfusion defect with either increased lung uptake (thallium-201) or LV dilation

    (d) *Stress echo*: echocardiographic wall motion abnormally (>2 segments) at low doses of dobutamine (≤10 mg/kg/min) or at a low heart rate (<120 beats/min)

Reprinted from Patel et al. [1] with permission from Elsevier and *J Am Coll Cardiol*

Table 6.2 CCS (Canadian Cardiovascular Society) grading of angina pectoris

Class I: Angina occurs with strenuous, rapid, or prolonged exertion

Class II: Slight limitation of ordinary activity. Angina occurs on walking more than 2 blocks on level ground and climbing more than 1 flight of ordinary stairs at a normal pace in normal conditions

Class III: Marked limitations of ordinary physical activity. Angina occurs on walking 1 or 2 blocks on level ground or climbing 1 flight of stairs in normal conditions and at a normal pace

Class IV: Inability to carry on any physical activity without discomfort. Anginal symptoms may be present at rest

Available on the Canadian Cardiovascular Society website at www.ccs.caand and reprinted from Campeau [2] with permission from Wolters Kluwer Health

Inappropriate PCI and What Not to Do by Guidelines

For ease, we will classify patients as:

- ACS patients
  - Stable patient: without any heart failure, unstable ventricular arrhythmias, recurrent or provocable ischemia, hemodynamic or electrical instability.
  - Unstable patient: presents with heart failure, unstable ventricular arrhythmias, recurrent or provocable ischemia, hemodynamic or electrical instability.
- Non-ACS patients

Acute Coronary Syndrome [ACS]-Inappropriate Criteria

- STEMI:
  - Asymptomatic stable patient after 12 h of symptom onset.
  - Asymptomatic stable patient with a normal EF and revascularization of a non-infarct-related artery during index hospitalization in a stable asymptomatic patient after successful treatment of the culprit artery by primary PCI or fibrinolysis.
- NSTEMI/UA – Nothing is inappropriate

Non-ACS

- CABG patients:
  - One or more stenosis in SVG.
    - Asymptomatic patient not on MMT with a low risk ST.
  - *Significant native vessel disease in non-bypassed arteries with all grafts patent.*
    - Asymptomatic patient with intermediate risk ST not on MMT or low risk ST.
    - *CSS Classes 1 and 2*: Low risk ST not on MMT (Table 6.2).
    - *CSS Classes 3 and 4* – Nothing is inappropriate (Table 6.2).
- Non-CABG patients:
  - *Asymptomatic*: <3 vessel CAD without involvement of proximal LAD.
    - Intermediate risk ST not on MMT or Low risk ST.
  - *CSS Classes 1 and 2*: <3 vessel CAD without involvement of proximal LAD and with low-risk ST *not* on MMT (Table 6.2).
  - *Irrespective of symptoms (even if CCS Class 3 or 4)* (Table 6.2):
    - CTO of 1 major coronary artery, without other coronary stenoses and low-risk ST and not on MMT.
    - <3 vessel CAD with borderline stenosis "50–60 %" and ST is equivocal or unavailable or FFR/IVUS not done or is not significant.

Method of Revascularization of Multivessel Coronary Artery Disease (PCI Inappropriate When Compared to CABG)

- Left main stenosis + intermediate to high CAD burden (3-vessel CAD or CTO or high SYNTAX score ≥33).
- 3-vessel CAD in a diabetic patient.

References

1. Patel MR, Dehmer GJ, Hirshfeld JW, Smith PK, Spertus JA. ACCF/SCAI/STS/AATS/AHA/ASNC/HFSA/SCCT 2012 appropriate use criteria for coronary revascularization focused update. J Am Coll Cardiol. 2012;59(9):857–81. PubMed PMID: 22296741.
2. Campeau L. Grading of angina pectoris. Circulation. 1976;54:5223.

Guide Catheter Selection

7

Anitha Rajamanickam and Samin Sharma

Optimal guide support is vital for successful interventions. An ideal guide catheter should have an atraumatic soft tip, excellent torque control, provide adequate support, and have a low surface frictional resistance to allow for good trackability of balloons and devices.

Guiding Catheter Layers

- The outer layer is polyurethane or polyethylene and is responsible for overall stiffness.
- The middle layer is composed of a wire matrix and is responsible for torque generation.
- The inner layer is composed of Teflon for smooth passage of balloons, stents, and devices (see Fig. 7.1).

Guide Selection

The guide catheter is usually firmly supported against the aortic wall opposite to the coronary sinus from which the artery arises. Selection is dependent on:

- *Side holes*
- *French sizes[Fr]*
- *Length*

A. Rajamanickam, MD (✉) • S. Sharma, MD, FACC
Department of Interventional Cardiology, Mount Sinai Hospital,
One Gustave Levy Place, Madison Avenue, New York, NY 10029, USA
e-mail: arajamanickam@gmail.com, Anitha.Rajamanickam@mountsinai.org;
Samin.sharma@mountsinai.org

© Springer-Verlag London 2014
A. Kini et al. (eds.), *Practical Manual of Interventional Cardiology*,
DOI 10.1007/978-1-4471-6581-1_7

Fig. 7.1 Guiding catheter layers

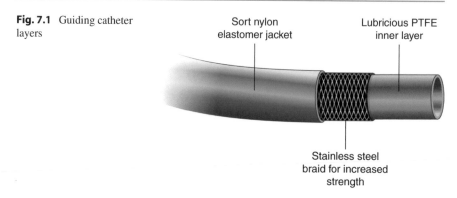

Sort nylon elastomer jacket

Lubricious PTFE inner layer

Stainless steel braid for increased strength

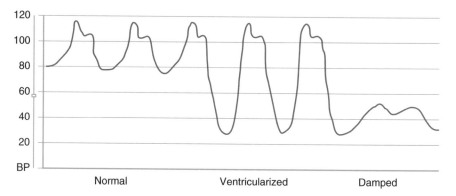

Normal   Ventricularized   Damped

Fig. 7.2 Ventricularization and damping

- *Type of curve – anatomy based*:
  - Size of the aortic root
  - Ostial origin and takeoff
- *Support*
- *Anomalous origin*

Step One: Side Holes Side holes prevent ventricularization [fall of diastolic pressure] or dampening [fall of both systolic and diastolic pressure] caused by engagement of guide in significant ostial lesions, misalignment of guides, during coronary spasm, or when a large Fr guide is used for engagement of a smaller coronary artery (see Fig. 7.2). See Table 7.1 for use, advantages, and disadvantages of side holes.

Step Two: French Sizes Ideally use the smallest diameter catheter feasible to minimize the risk of arterial damage (Fig. 7.3). Larger French catheters have the advantage of improved opacification, better guide support and allow for pressure

Table 7.1 Side holes in guide catheters: use, advantages, and disadvantages

Advantages	Disadvantages
Maintains coronary artery perfusion	False sense of security as it monitors aortic not coronary pressure
	Suboptimal opacification
	Increase in contrast volume

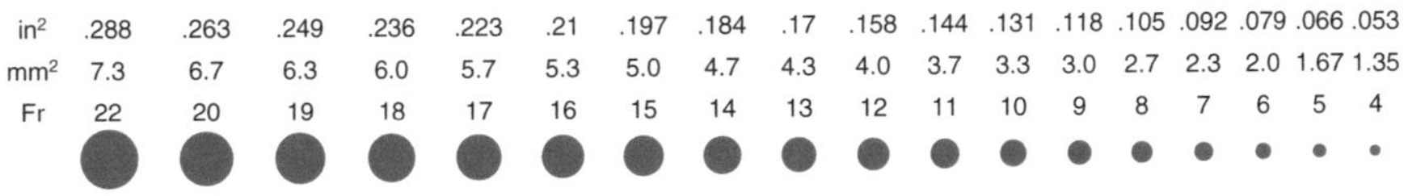

in²	.288	.263	.249	.236	.223	.21	.197	.184	.17	.158	.144	.131	.118	.105	.092	.079	.066	.053
mm²	7.3	6.7	6.3	6.0	5.7	5.3	5.0	4.7	4.3	4.0	3.7	3.3	3.0	2.7	2.3	2.0	1.67	1.35
Fr	22	20	19	18	17	16	15	14	13	12	11	10	9	8	7	6	5	4

Fig. 7.3 French sizes

monitoring but increase the risk of ostial trauma, vascular complications, and contrast nephropathy.

- Usually 6 Fr guides will suffice for most interventions.
- 7 Fr: Two-stent strategy for bifurcation lesions [modified T technique, SKS technique, V technique] and rotational atherectomy burr of 2 mm.
- 8 Fr: Rotational atherectomy burr of 2.15 or 2.25 mm.

Step Three: Guide Length

- Regular 110 cm guides will suffice for most coronary interventions.
- Long saphenous vein graft (SVG) or internal mammary artery (IMA) grafts interventions may require the use of short 80 or 90 cm guides.

Step Four: Support The most commonly used guides are the Judkins (JL/JR), Amplatz (AL/AR), Voda(VL), internal mammary (IM), and extra backup (EBU). Support is either passive or active.

- *Passive support:* Depends on the guide design, stiffness and its backup support against the opposite aortic wall or aortocoronary sinus.
- *Active support:* Manipulation of the guide to conform with the aortic root or deep engagement of the guide into the coronary arteries provides active support for interventions.

Other Maneuvers to Improve Support

- Types of guides for support:
  - Left : EBU/XB > VL > JL
  - Right : AL > AR/IM > JR

Table 7.2 Size of aortic root

Size	Left	Right
Normal (3.5–4 cm)	VL 3.5	IM, FR, AR2, AL 0.75
Large (>4 cm)	VL 4, VL 4.5	IM, AL 1, AL 2
Small (<3.5 cm)	VL 3	IM, FR

- Use of a long sheath
- Increasing guide size
- Buddy wire
- Anchoring balloon
- GuideLiner and mother-in-child techniques

Step Five: Catheter Curve Select curve styles optimal for a given anatomical configuration (Table 7.2).

Our first go to guide is VL for the left interventions, IM for the right interventions, and IM, AL0.75, AL1, or AR2 for SVG interventions.

Know Your Normal Ostial Origin

- Left main usually arises anterior, inferior, and leftward from the left coronary sinus:
    - LAD usually arises in an anteriorly and superiorly from the left main.
    - LCX usually arises posteriorly and inferiorly from the left main.
- RCA usually arises anteriorly from the right aortic cusp.
- SVGs usually arise anteriorly from the aorta.

Actual Ostial Origin

Coronary ostial location (see Fig. 7.4 and Table 7.3):

- High
- Low
- Anterior
- Posterior

Coronary ostial orientation:

- Superior
- Horizontal
- Inferior
- Shepherd's crook (RCAs only)

Fig. 7.4 Ostial origins of the coronary arteries

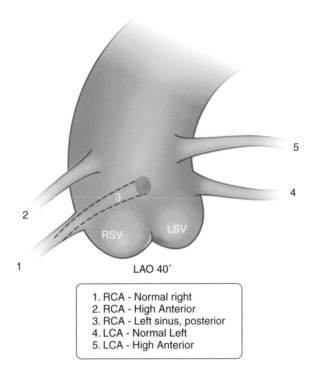

Cornary artery variations

2

3

RSV   LSV

1

LAO 40°

1. RCA - Normal right
2. RCA - High Anterior
3. RCA - Left sinus, posterior
4. LCA - Normal Left
5. LCA - High Anterior

5

4

Table 7.3 Guide selection depending on origin of the coronary ostia

Origin	Left coronary	Right coronary
Anterior	Not applicable	NoTo, 3DRC, AR2 or AL0.75(dilated aortic root)
Shepherd's crook	Not applicable	SCR, HS, IMA
Short left main	FL, FCL, VL3	Not applicable
Long left main	VL4	Not applicable

Catheter Selection for Anomalous Right Coronary Arteries

In the LAO view draw an imaginary line at the upper edge of the bulge which marks the plane dividing the aortic sinuses from the ascending aorta. A similar line drawn along the lower edge of this bulge divides the aortic cusps from the ventricular outflow tract. Finally, a line is drawn along the long axis of the ascending aorta intersecting the sinus aortic and aorto-ventricular planes perpendicularly. The origin of the anomalous vessel is described based on its location in relation to these landmarks (see Fig. 7.5 and Table 7.4). Please refer to Fig. 7.6 for the different guide catheter shapes, sizing, and unique characteristics.

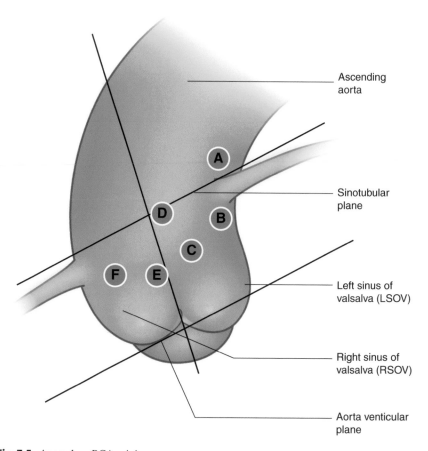

Fig. 7.5 Anomalous RCA origins

Table 7.4 Catheter selection for anomalous right coronary arteries

Type	Origin	First choice	Second choice
From left cusp			
A	From the aorta above the sinotubular plane	FL3	FCL3
B	Just below the ostium of the left coronary artery	FCL 3	FCL 3.5,VL3.5
C	Below the sinotubular plane between the midline and the origin of the left coronary artery	VL 3.5	FCL3.5
D	Origin near the midline	AL1	AL .75, AL2, AL3
From right cusp			
E	Origin near the midline	AR2	AR 1
F	Anterior origin	3D RC	AR2,AR1

Left coronary guides

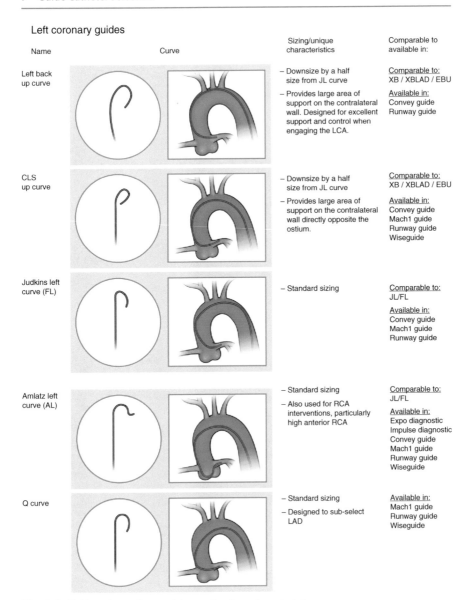

Name	Curve	Sizing/unique characteristics	Comparable to available in:
Left back up curve		– Downsize by a half size from JL curve – Provides large area of support on the contralateral wall. Designed for excellent support and control when engaging the LCA.	Comparable to: XB / XBLAD / EBU Available in: Convey guide Runway guide
CLS up curve		– Downsize by a half size from JL curve – Provides large area of support on the contralateral wall directly opposite the ostium.	Comparable to: XB / XBLAD / EBU Available in: Convey guide Mach1 guide Runway guide Wiseguide
Judkins left curve (FL)		– Standard sizing	Comparable to: JL/FL Available in: Convey guide Mach1 guide Runway guide
Amlatz left curve (AL)		– Standard sizing – Also used for RCA interventions, particularly high anterior RCA	Comparable to: JL/FL Available in: Expo diagnostic Impulse diagnostic Convey guide Mach1 guide Runway guide Wiseguide
Q curve		– Standard sizing – Designed to sub-select LAD	Available in: Mach1 guide Runway guide Wiseguide

Fig. 7.6   Guide catheter shapes, sizing, and unique characteristics

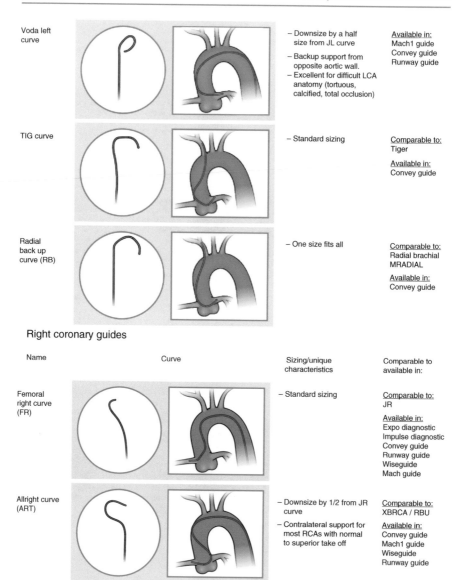

Voda left curve		– Downsize by a half size from JL curve – Backup support from opposite aortic wall. – Excellent for difficult LCA anatomy (tortuous, calcified, total occlusion)	Available in: Mach1 guide Convey guide Runway guide
TIG curve		– Standard sizing	Comparable to: Tiger Available in: Convey guide
Radial back up curve (RB)		– One size fits all	Comparable to: Radial brachial MRADIAL Available in: Convey guide

Right coronary guides

Name	Curve	Sizing/unique characteristics	Comparable to available in:
Femoral right curve (FR)		– Standard sizing	Comparable to: JR Available in: Expo diagnostic Impulse diagnostic Convey guide Runway guide Wiseguide Mach guide
Allright curve (ART)		– Downsize by 1/2 from JR curve – Contralateral support for most RCAs with normal to superior take off	Comparable to: XBRCA / RBU Available in: Convey guide Mach1 guide Wiseguide Runway guide

Fig. 7.6 (continued)

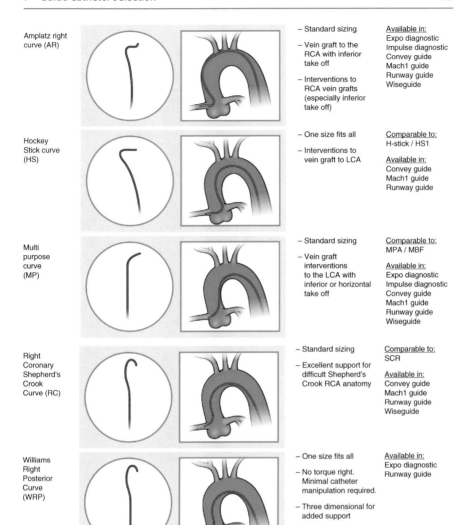

Amplatz right curve (AR)	– Standard sizing – Vein graft to the RCA with inferior take off – Interventions to RCA vein grafts (especially inferior take off)	Available in: Expo diagnostic Impulse diagnostic Convey guide Mach1 guide Runway guide Wiseguide
Hockey Stick curve (HS)	– One size fits all – Interventions to vein graft to LCA	Comparable to: H-stick / HS1 Available in: Convey guide Mach1 guide Runway guide
Multi purpose curve (MP)	– Standard sizing – Vein graft interventions to the LCA with inferior or horizontal take off	Comparable to: MPA / MBF Available in: Expo diagnostic Impulse diagnostic Convey guide Mach1 guide Runway guide Wiseguide
Right Coronary Shepherd's Crook Curve (RC)	– Standard sizing – Excellent support for difficult Shepherd's Crook RCA anatomy	Comparable to: SCR Available in: Convey guide Mach1 guide Runway guide Wiseguide
Williams Right Posterior Curve (WRP)	– One size fits all – No torque right. Minimal catheter manipulation required. – Three dimensional for added support	Available in: Expo diagnostic Runway guide

Fig. 7.6   (continued)

Bypass graft guides

Name	Curve	Sizing/unique characteristics	
Internal Mammary Curve (IM)	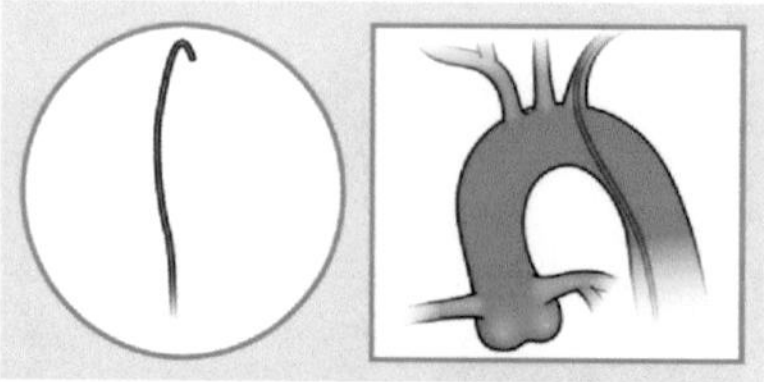	–One size fits all –Incorporates a large radius primary curve designed to ease device passage. –Provides contralateral support from the subclavian artery	Available in: Expo diagnostic Impulse diagnostic Convey guide Mach 1 guide Runway guide Wiseguide
Left Coronary Bypass Curve (LCB)	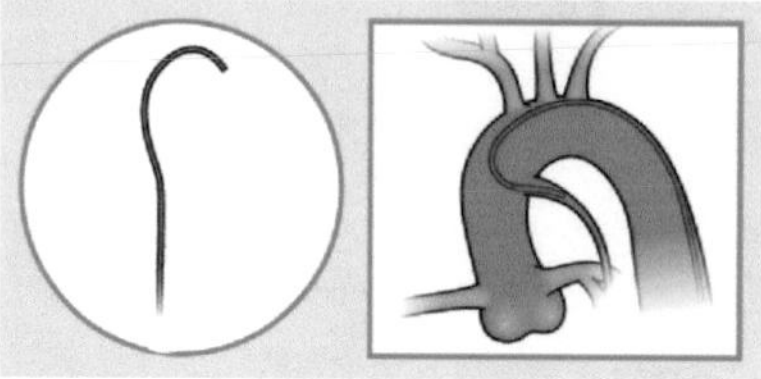	–One size fits all –Similar to JR and HS. –Useful for vein grafts to the LCA with horizontal or slightly superior take off	Available in: Expo diagnostic Convey guiding Mach1 guide Runway guide Wiseguide

Fig. 7.6 (continued)

Guidewire Properties and Selection

8

Christopher J. Varughese, Anitha Rajamanickam,
and Samin Sharma

The cornerstone to a successful percutaneous coronary intervention involves the appropriate selection of a coronary guidewire that can support and enable easy navigation of coronary devices through various coronary anatomies. The basic construct of the coronary guidewire has the following functions:

- To track through the vessel
- To access the lesion
- To cross the lesion atraumatically
- To provide support for interventional devices

While there are numerous guidewires available, the key characteristics of the guidewire remain consistent across manufacturers.

Structure of the Guidewire

There are three main components of the guidewire (see Fig. 8.1):

- Core
- Tip
- Covering

C.J. Varughese, MD • A. Rajamanickam, MD • S. Sharma, MD, FACC (✉)
Department of Interventional Cardiology, Mount Sinai Hospital,
One Gustave Levy Place, Madison Avenue, New York, NY 10029, USA
e-mail: cvarughese@gmail.com; arajamanickam@gmail.com,
Anitha.Rajamanickam@mountsinai.org; Samin.sharma@mountsinai.org

© Springer-Verlag London 2014
A. Kini et al. (eds.), *Practical Manual of Interventional Cardiology*,
DOI 10.1007/978-1-4471-6581-1_8

Fig. 8.1 Guidewire structure
(Courtesy of Abbott Vascular.
©2014 Abbott. All Rights
Reserved)

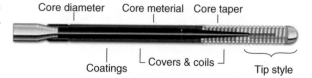

Core

The Core is the innermost part of the guidewire, and extends through the shaft of the wire from the proximal to the distal end where it begins to taper. The diameter of the core influences the flexibility, support, and torque, while the core material affects the steering, trackability, in addition to flexibility and support.

- *Core Material*
  - *Stainless steel (SS):*
    - *Strengths*: provide optimal support, transmission of force, torque characteristics, and good shapeability
    - *Weakness*: more susceptible to kinking
  - Nitinol, a super-elastic alloy of nickel and titanium with excellent resiliency and kink resistance:
    - *Strengths*: It provides excellent flexibility and steerability and is more durable than stainless steel. Due to its ability to resist deformation, it is often used for treatment of multiple lesions and tortuous anatomy.
    - *Weakness*: less torqueability than SS.
- *Core diameter*
  The diameter of the core influences the performance of the wire. A larger wire improves support and allows for 1:1 torque response, while smaller diameters have the opposite effect and enhance flexibility of the wire.
- *Core taper*
  The core of the guidewire is tapered along its length. The taper may be continuous or segmental and variable in length. Shorter tapers and smaller numbers of widely spaced gradual tapers enhance the support and transmission of push force, while longer tapers and larger numbers of more segmental tapering enhance the flexibility.

Tip

The tip refers to the distal end of the guidewire. There are two types of tips. The tip could be covered with coils (spring-tip guidewires) or polymer (polymer-tip guidewires):

- *Core to tip design*
  The most commonly used wires have a one-piece core where the core extends all the way to the tip with a variable taper. These wires are engineered to possess precise steering and tip control and a soft tip.
- *Two-piece or shaping ribbon*
  The core stops just before the distal tip. A shaping ribbon (a small piece of metal) bridges the gap between the end of the core and the distal tip which allows for a very flexible, soft, atraumatic tip with easy shaping and good shape retention. However, compared to other designs these wires have less reliable torque control and a higher likelihood to prolapse.

Covering

To maintain the overall diameter of 0.014 in., all guidewires have a specific surface coating:

- *Coils*
  Stainless steel coils are the outer wire components. In an outer coil design, coils are placed over the tapered core and tip of the wire as opposed to the tip coil design (shaping ribbon); the tip alone is covered with coils. These coils add flexibility to the distal part of the wire as well as support, steering, trackability and visibility. Visibility of the wire tip is provided by radiopaque platinum coils that are usually placed at the distal tip (usually 2–3 cms long). Coils placed on the working length of the wire are referred to as intermediate coils.
- *Covers*
  Some wires have polymer or plastic covering over the tapered wire core instead of outer coils. The use of polymer or plastic covering provides the wire with lubricity and enables smooth tracking through tortuous anatomy.
- *Coating*
  The coating refers to the outer covering that keeps the overall diameter consistent and influences the wire performance. The type and length of coating may vary and are most often applied to the distal 30 cm of the wire. Two types of coatings are used:
  - *Hydrophilic coatings* attract water and are applied along the entire length of the wire including the tip coils. When dry, the coating is solid, thin and non-slippery solid. Upon contact with liquids, the coating becomes a slippery "waxlike" surface that reduces friction and increases trackability. While providing for a lubricous low-friction motion inside the vessel, these wires should be utilized judiciously as they carry the risk of subintimal penetration, dissection, and perforation of the coronary artery.
  - *Hydrophobic coatings* are silicone-based coatings which repel water. It is applied to the working length wire except for the distal tip. The silicone coating has higher-friction and is more stable inside the vessel and is not activated by liquids.

Classification of Guidewires

The classification of guidewires can be broken down into three categories:

- *Tip flexibility*
- *Device support*
- *Coating type*

Guidewire Manipulation

Shaping the Wire Tip Shape the tip using the shaping needle that comes with the wire or the introducer needle. Usually a simple J curve with a distal bend that approximates the vessel diameter will allow the guidewire to track through the vessel. Careful manipulation of the guidewire during shaping is warranted to avoid damaging the structure and solidity of the guidewire (Fig. 8.2).

Steering When steering the wire through the vessel, the wire should be gently advanced and pass smoothly through the stenosis. Forceful manipulation can disrupt plaque and cause thrombus formation and acute occlusion. While advancing the guidewire, a repeated rotation of 180° in clockwise and counterclockwise directions will reduce the likelihood of subselection of unwanted small branches. One should avoid a complete 360° rotation as this may result in tip fracture or entanglement with a second wire. The wire tip should be placed as distally as possible, so the stiff part of the wire is across the lesion where the stent and other interventional devices are to be tracked.

Wiring the LAD The best initial view to enter the LAD is the left anterior oblique (LAO) caudal view (spider view). Once the wire has been advanced far enough, change to the right anterior oblique (RAO) cranial view so the wire can be traversed to mid and then distal LAD.

Wiring the LCX For LCX interventions, a broader tip is warranted to successfully enter the LCX and a smaller curve to cross the obtuse marginal.

Wiring the RCA If the origin of the RCA is relatively normal, a conventional soft wire with good steerability to avoid side branches is chosen first.

Selection of Guidewires

The selection of a guidewire should be primarily determined by vessel morphology, lesion morphology, and device properties (see Fig. 8.3).

Guidewires for Standard Lesion Morphology A standard lesion is defined by the absence of complex characteristics (i.e., heavy calcification, tortuous segments, and total occlusions). A "workhorse or frontline" wire is most suitable for standard lesions (Table 8.1). The workhorse wire, which accounts for about 70 % of all coronary wires used, is a floppy wire with atraumatic tip which provides low to moderate support.

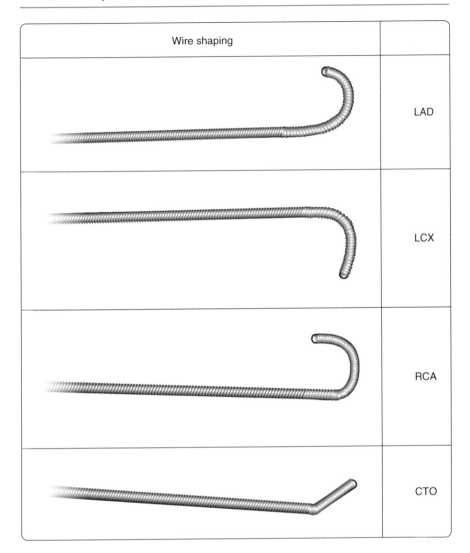

Wire shaping	
	LAD
	LCX
	RCA
	CTO

Fig. 8.2 Shaping of the guidewire

The preferred workhorse wire at the Mount Sinai Cardiac Catheterization Laboratory is currently the Terumo Runthrough NS wire. Unlike its stainless steel wire predecessors (Balance Middleweight and Prowater wires), it has a unique core design with the main shaft core of stainless steel and a distal core of nitinol alloy which extends into a nitinol shaping ribbon. The distal tip is hydrophilic coated. These properties give it a better steerability which allows for easier navigation through difficult angulated lesions.

Guidewires for Chronic Total Occlusions For the more complex lesions, particularly chronic total occlusions (CTO), a stiffer wire with increasing support may be required (see Tables 8.2 and 8.3).

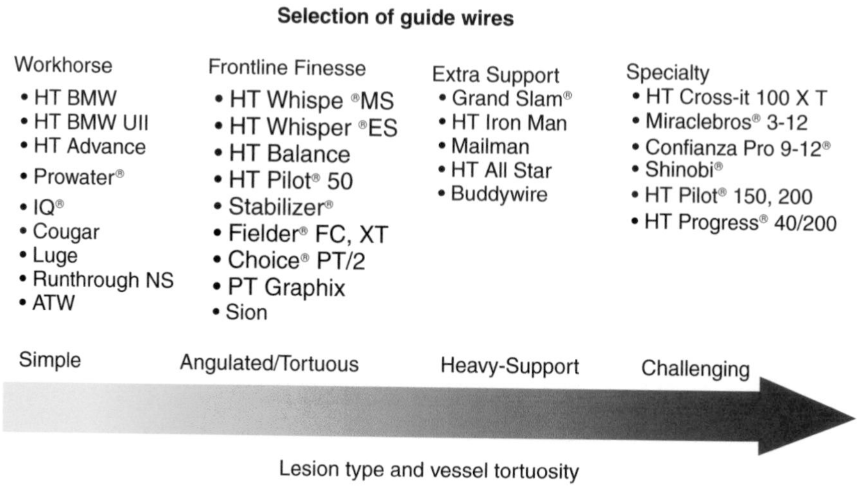

Selection of guide wires

Workhorse	Frontline Finesse	Extra Support	Specialty
• HT BMW	• HT Whispe ®MS	• Grand Slam®	• HT Cross-it 100 X T
• HT BMW UII	• HT Whisper ®ES	• HT Iron Man	• Miraclebros® 3-12
• HT Advance	• HT Balance	• Mailman	• Confianza Pro 9-12®
• Prowater®	• HT Pilot® 50	• HT All Star	• Shinobi®
• IQ®	• Stabilizer®	• Buddywire	• HT Pilot® 150, 200
• Cougar	• Fielder® FC, XT		• HT Progress® 40/200
• Luge	• Choice® PT/2		
• Runthrough NS	• PT Graphix		
• ATW	• Sion		

Simple   Angulated/Tortuous   Heavy-Support   Challenging

Lesion type and vessel tortuosity

Fig. 8.3 Selection of a guidewire by morphology and support (Courtesy of Abbott Vascular. ©2014 Abbott. All Rights Reserved)

Table 8.1 Workhorse wires

Guidewire	Tip load (g)	Radiopaque length (cm)	Tip diameter	Polymer cover	Coating
Runthrough NS	1	3	0.014	Full	Hydrophilic
Balance Middleweight wire	0.8	3	0.014	None	Hydrophilic
Whisper ES	1.2	3	0.014	Full	Hydrophilic

Table 8.2 CTO wires by name

Guidewire	Tip load	Radiopaque length	Tip diameter	Polymer cover	Coating
Fielder	3.7	3	0.014	Full	Hydrophilic
Fielder FC	1.6	3	0.014	Full	Hydrophilic
Fielder XT	1.2	16	0.009	Full	Hydrophilic
MiracleBros 3	3.9	11	0.0125	None	Hydrophobic
MiracleBros 4.5	4.4	11	0.0125	None	Hydrophobic
MiracleBros 6	8.8	11	0.0125	None	Hydrophobic
MiracleBros 12	13	11	0.0125	None	Hydrophobic
Confianza 9	8.6	20	0.009	None	Hydrophobic
Confianza PRO 9	9.3	20	0.009	None	Hybrid
Confianza PRO 12	12.4	20	0.009	None	Hybrid
PROGRESS 40	4.8	3	0.012	Tip only	Hydrophilic
PROGRESS 80	9.7	3	0.012	Tip only	Hydrophilic
PROGRESS 120	13.9	3	0.012	Tip only	Hydrophilic

Table 8.2 (continued)

Guidewire	Tip load	Radiopaque length	Tip diameter	Polymer cover	Coating
PROGRESS 140 T	12.5	3	0.0105	Tip only	Hydrophilic
PROGRESS 200 T	13.3	3	0.009	Tip only	Hydrophilic
HT PILOT 200	4.1	3	0.014	Full	Hydrophilic
HT PILOT 150	2.7	3	0.014	Full	Hydrophilic
HT PILOT 50	1.5	3	0.014	Full	Hydrophilic

Table 8.3 CTO wires [by tip load]

Guidewire	Tip load	Radiopaque length	Tip diameter	Polymer cover	Coating
Fielder XT	1.2	16	0.009	Full	Hydrophilic
HT PILOT 50	1.5	3	0.014	Full	Hydrophilic
FIELDER FC	1.6	3	0.014	Full	Hydrophilic
HT PILOT 150	2.7	3	0.014	Full	Hydrophilic
Fielder	3.7	3	0.014	Full	Hydrophilic
MiracleBros 3	3.9	11	0.0125	None	Hydrophobic
HT PILOT 200	4.1	3	0.014	Full	Hydrophilic
MiracleBros 4.5	4.4	11	0.0125	None	Hydrophobic
PROGRESS 40	4.8	3	0.012	Tip only	Hydrophilic
Confianza 9	8.6	20	0.009	None	Hydrophobic
MiracleBros 6	8.8	11	0.0125	None	Hydrophobic
Confianza PRO 9	9.3	20	0.009	None	Hybrid
PROGRESS 80	9.7	3	0.012	Tip only	Hydrophilic
Confianza PRO 12	12.4	20	0.009	None	Hybrid
PROGRESS 140 T	12.5	3	0.0105	Tip only	Hydrophilic
MiracleBros 12	13	11	0.0125	None	Hydrophobic
PROGRESS 200 T	13.3	3	0.009	Tip only	Hydrophilic
PROGRESS 120	13.9	3	0.012	Tip only	Hydrophilic

Technical Tips

Better Torque Control   When a wire is more difficult to manipulate after it passes through too many curves, advancement of the balloon catheter to near the wire tip will improve wire support, torque control, and steerability. Other options include use of stiffer wire or hydrophilic wires, which are very sleek and kink resistant. However, since they are so smooth, the operator has little tactile feedback; they can easily enter subintimally or cause distal perforation if inadvertently advanced into a small and short branch. So, when manipulating a hydrophilic wire, always watch the distal tip, to avoid inadvertent migration and perforation.

Wire Prolapsing When navigating a curve in order to enter an artery (e.g., from the LM into the LCX), a floppy wire may keep prolapsing into a unintended artery (e.g., LAD). The reason is the abrupt transition between the short tip and the main shaft. The way to resolve this is to change to a wire with a gradually tapered core so that as the tip is deeply advanced, it stabilizes the wire and the stiffer shaft can negotiate the angle better, without prolapsing into an unintended area (or LAD). Once the soft part of the tip passes the acute corner, torque the wire slowly while advancing the wire. The rotational energy will advance the wire distally.

Enter the LCX without changing the wire. When navigating the LM in order to enter a sharp bifurcation of the LCX, perform the following maneuver.

• Apply clockwise torque on the guide so its tip will point toward the LCX ostium, especially if the LM is short.
• Ask the patient to take a deep breath that elongates the heart and straightens the angle between the LM and LCX. In this short window of opportunity, advance the wire into the LCX. If this is unsuccessful, then remove the wire and shape the tip to conform with the entry angle of the LM and LCX.

Advancing a Wire Through Severely Angulated Segment By Pulling It Back In rare instances, a wire has to enter a very severely angulated segment. The tip of the wire should be curved to form a large diameter curve. Once the tip enters the branch, the wire is withdrawn to prolapse the tip into the intended branch. Then rotate the wire toward the main lumen, clockwise if the tip was pointing toward the left of the patient and counterclockwise if the tip was pointing toward the right of the patient. If there is enough stiff segment inside the side branch (not just the soft tip), then the wire will advance further, without prolapsing back (Fig. 4.1).

Directing the Wire When Navigating the LAD In case of navigating the LAD, at first at the LAO caudal view, the wire should point to the right on the screen. The left is toward the diagonal. Once inside the proximal segment, the better view is the RAO or LAO cranial view. Here the wire should move downward. Any stray to the left will point to the diagonal and to the right will point to the septals.

Crossing a Stent If a stent needs to be re-crossed, the tip of the guidewire should be curved well into a wide J and the whole wire can be advanced while being rotated. This maneuver will help to avoid the inadvertent migration of the tip of the catheter under a strut. If there is subtle resistance, then wire exit through or behind the struts is suspected. If the stented area has sudden acute thrombosis and a curved tip fails to cross the stent, then an intermediate wire with a mildly bent tip can be manipulated to cross the stent. Try to have the pictures of the segments in two orthogonal views so the wire can be advanced inside the lumen as best as possible.

Assessment of Lesion Severity (Intravascular Ultrasound, Optical Coherence Tomography, NIRS, and Beyond)

Sadik Raja Panwar, Anitha Rajamanickam, and Annapoorna Kini

Intravascular Ultrasound (IVUS)

IVUS is one of the new tools in our interventional armamentarium which is catheter based miniature ultrasound device which enables us to view the artery from inside. The oscillatory movement (expansion and contraction) of a piezoelectric transducer (crystal) in the IVUS when electrically excited produces sound waves which propagate through the different tissues and are reflected according to the acoustic properties of the tissue it travels through. These reflected sound waves are then transcribed into a three dimensional gray scale image.

Indications

- To determine lumen area, lesion complexity (e.g., plaque burden, calcification), and lesion length, especially in bifurcations lesions.
- To determine the severity of angiographically intermediate left main disease.
- To determine stent apposition, lesion coverage, and edge dissection post stent deployment.
  - To optimize stent expansion and prevent stent thrombosis or restenosis.
  - To assess for adequate stent expansion, especially in cases of in-stent restenosis and stent thrombosis.
  - To assess coronary vasculopathy in transplanted hearts.

S.R. Panwar, MD (✉) • A. Rajamanickam, MD • A. Kini, MD, MRCP, FACC
Department of Interventional Cardiology, Mount Sinai Hospital,
One Gustave Levy Place, Madison Avenue, New York, NY 10029, USA
e-mail: drsrpanwar@gmail.com; arajamanickam@gmail.com,
Anitha.Rajamanickam@mountsinai.org; Annapoorna.kini@mountsinai.org

© Springer-Verlag London 2014
A. Kini et al. (eds.), *Practical Manual of Interventional Cardiology*,
DOI 10.1007/978-1-4471-6581-1_9

How it works

- IVUS catheters can either be a mechanical system rotating a single transducer or a multitransducer array that is activated sequentially to produce an image.
- Ultrasound waves from the IVUS catheter are reflected by the tissue to create a 360° tomographic image of the vessel wall from the intima to the media.
- IVUS resolution is 100–200 μm, showing the lumen–intima interface and, to a lesser degree, the interface between the media and intima.
- Unlike optical coherence tomography (OCT) imaging, IVUS does not require blood to be cleared from the vessel.

Limits

- Gives no physiologic evaluation of lesion severity.
- In the absence of FFR, it can be used to decide whether to stent an intermediate lesion, but the specificity of IVUS for obstructive lesions is suboptimal.
- May be difficult to pass the catheter across highly stenotic lesions or tortuous vessels.

Equipment and practical aspects

- ≥5F sheath.
- Heparin or bivalirudin for ACT >250 s.
- Engage target vessel and wire the lesion.
- Flush the IVUS catheter with saline.
- Administer 200 μg of intracoronary nitroglycerin.
- The blood vessel does not have to be cleared of blood for imaging to occur.
- Automated mechanical pullback is the best choice for precise imaging.
- Once the catheter pullback is completed, IVUS computer software can be used to determine minimal luminal area (MLA) of the lesion (Table 9.1).

Detailed discussion Interobserver variability in determining the severity of stenosis angiographically has been consistently demonstrated [1, 2]. IVUS provides more objective measurement of vessel size and lesion length and quality (Figs. 9.1, 9.2, 9.3, and 9.4), and can guide device selection (e.g., the need for rotablation or the use of a longer stent). IVUS-guided PCI leads to greater acute vessel gain, as well as better outcomes with respect to BMS restenosis and DES thrombosis [3, 4]. In our experience, IVUS

Table 9.1 IVUS numbers to remember

ACT >250 ms before IVUS catheter insertion
Left main MLA >6 mm^2 or non-left main MLA ≥4 mm^2, safe to defer stenting
MLA <4 mm^2 ≠ FFR <0.80, *but, in the absence of FFR:*
MLA <3 mm^2 in the proximal LAD correlates with FFR <0.80
MLA <2.75 mm^2 in the LAD after the second diagonal branch
MLA <2.4 mm^2 for non-LAD vessels may predict FFR <0.80
Intimal thickness >0.5 mm consistent with transplant coronary vasculopathy

Fig. 9.1 Normal coronary
artery

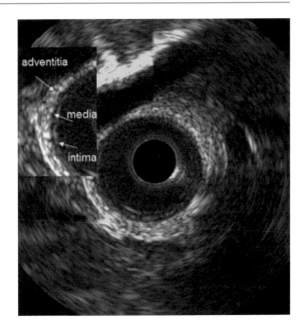

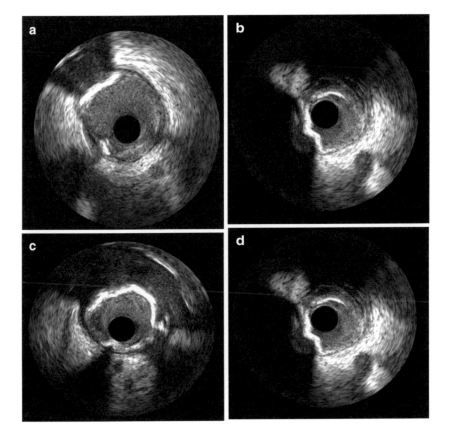

Fig. 9.2 Calcified plaque (hyperechoic) on IVUS

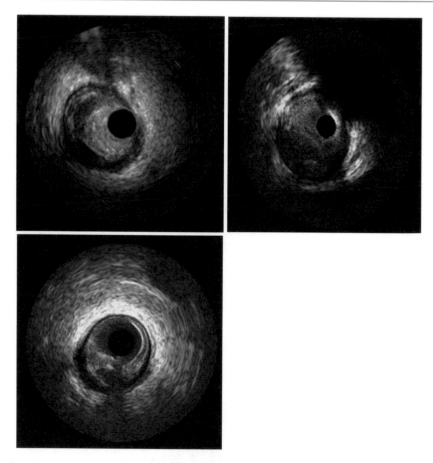

Fig. 9.3 Lipid pool (echolucent area within plaque) on IVUS

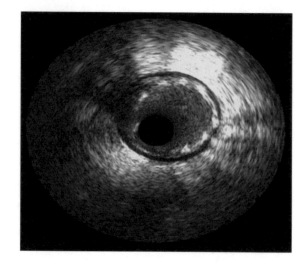

Fig. 9.4 Stented plaque by
IVUS

evaluation of lesion length and quality can also reduce contrast use and ensure adequate lesion coverage. In the transplanted heart, IVUS is a sensitive tool for detection of coronary artery vasculopathy, typically defined as intimal thickness >0.5 mm. As IUS does not provide physiological assessment, FFR is the best modality to determine if an angiographically indeterminate lesion requires percutaneous intervention (PCI). The hemodynamic significance of a lesion depends on numerous variables (e.g., target vessel stenosis severity, lesion length, area of the viable myocardium supplied by the vessel), which are reflected by FFR, but are unaccounted for by IVUS. A rough guide to IVUS measurements that correlate to hemodynamically significant stenoses is listed in Table 9.1 [5, 6]. As FFR has not been validated in instent restenosis, IVUS may be used to guide therapy in angiographically indeterminate lesions (MLA of the left main >6 mm^2 or MLA ≥4 mm^2 in a non-left main vessel is the cuttoff criteria used for defining non-ischemic intermediate lesions in which stenting is safely deferred).

Optical Coherence Tomography (OCT)

Optical coherence tomography (OCT) is an newer intravascular imaging technology for evaluating the cross-sectional and three-dimensional (3D) microstructure of blood vessels at a resolution of approximately 10 μm. The underlying principle of OCT is based on the concept that structural information of the coronary vessel can be obtained by measuring the delay time of optical echoes reflected or backscattered from subsurface structures in biological tissues, OCT light is in the near-infrared (NIR) range, typically with wavelengths of approximately 1.3 μm, which are not visible to the human eye (Table 9.2). Because of its higher resolution than intravascular ultrasound (IVUS), OCT can characterize the superficial structure of the vessel wall in greater detail (Table 9.2). OCT cannot image through blood because blood attenuates light before it reaches the arterial wall. As a result, OCT images are acquired as blood is flushed from the field of view.

Table 9.2 Physical characteristics of FD-OCT versus IVUS

	FD-OCT	IVUS
Radiation type	Light	Ultrasound
Wavelength, μm	1.3	35–80
Frequency	20–45 MHz	190 THz
Resolution, μm	10–40	100–150
Penetration depth, mm	1–3	4–10
Field-of-view diameter, mm	15	7–10
Frame rate, frames/s	100	30
Pullback speed, mm/s	20	0.5–1
Plaque characterization	Yes	Yes
Fibrous cap measurement	Yes	No
Vessel remodeling	No	Yes
Blood removal required	Yes	No

How it works

- Infrared light emitted from an optical fiber in the imaging catheter is reflected by the coronary vessel tissue, allowing for characterization of vessel wall.
- Resolution is 10–20 μm, but tissue penetration is only 1–2 mm.

Limits

- Tissue penetration is limited, allowing for imaging of only the superficial structures.
- Left main and ostial lesions are not satisfactorily imaged as the blood cannot be cleared adequately.

Indications

- Assessment of plaque morphology (e.g., plaque erosion in ACS) (Figs. 9.5 and 9.6)
  - To determine stent apposition, lesion coverage, and edge dissection (Fig. 9.6)
  - To optimize stent expansion to prevent stent thrombosis or restenosis
  - To assess for adequate stent expansion, especially in cases of in-stent restenosis and stent thrombosis

Equipment and practical aspects

- ≥6F sheath.
- Heparin or bivalirudin for ACT >250 s.
- Engage target vessel and wire the lesion.

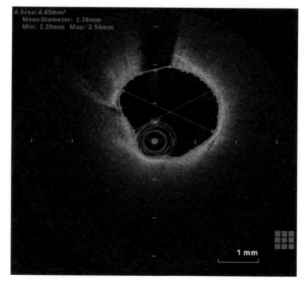

Fig. 9.5 OCT of an LAD lesion. Note the OCT catheter at 7 o'clock. In addition to highly accurate measurements of vessel diameter, lesion qualities can be assessed with greater accuracy than with IVUS

- Open the OCT catheter from packaging and flush the OCT catheter with attached 3 cc syringe using undiluted contrast to purge air from the catheter.
- Connect the catheter to the controller unit with a click.
- Administer 200 µg of intracoronary nitroglycerin.
- Back-load the guidewire through the OCT catheter and advance the distal tip of the catheter past the region of interest.
- Set the power injector according to the manufacturer's instructions (typically at least 3 cc/sec for a total volume of 12 cc for RCA and 4 cc/sec for a total volume of 14 cc for left coronaries (no more than 450 PSI).
- Check catheter position with a test injection.
- Once assured of position, activate the imaging catheter and inject 100 % contrast through the power injector.

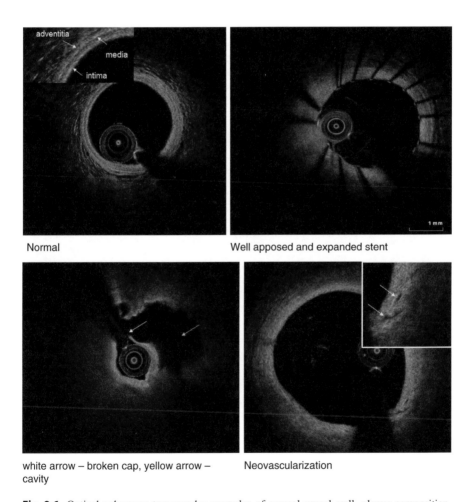

Normal   Well apposed and expanded stent

white arrow – broken cap, yellow arrow –   Neovascularization
cavity

Fig. 9.6 Optical coherence tomography examples of normal vessel wall, plaque composition, thrombus, and findings after coronary stenting

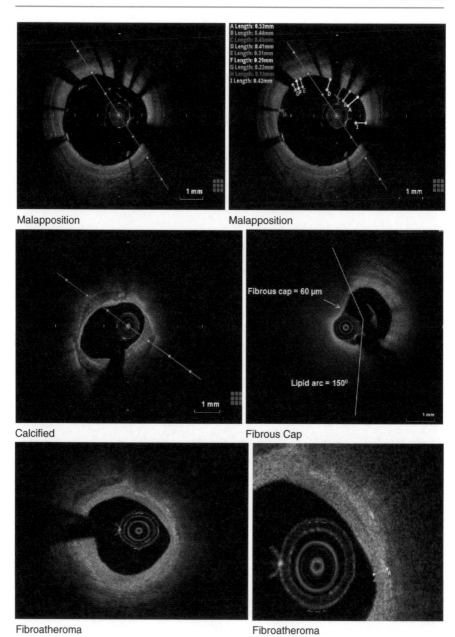

Fig. 9.6 (continued)

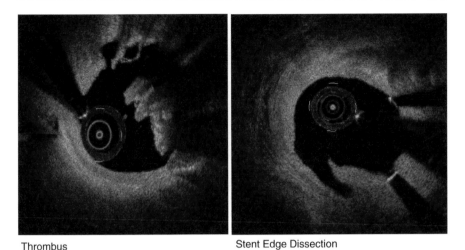

Thrombus   Stent Edge Dissection

Fig. 9.6 (continued)

Detailed discussion OCT's high resolution means it is more sensitive than IVUS for plaque characterization and vessel anatomy (Figs. 9.5 and 9.6). At present, OCT is primarily a research tool, though there are data to suggest that adjunctive use of OCT in PCI may lead to better outcomes and can guide decision making in ACS [7, 8]. Nonetheless, a routine role for OCT in PCI has yet to be determined.

Near-Infrared Spectroscopy (NIRS)–Intravascular Ultrasound (IVUS) Imaging

Indications The Infraredx TVC Imaging System™ is intended for the detection of lipid core-containing plaques (LCPs) using near-infrared spectroscopy (NIRS) and intravascular ultrasound (IVUS) examination of the coronary arteries. The combination of NIRS with IVUS in a single catheter combines the benefit of NIRS to the benefits of IVUS.

How it works The TVC Imaging System utilizes diffuse reflectance near-infrared spectroscopy (NIRS), a classic method of analytical chemistry, to characterize the plaque for lipid content [1]. Diffuse reflectance spectroscopy requires scattering and absorption at different wavelengths of the light by the tissue. First, the combination

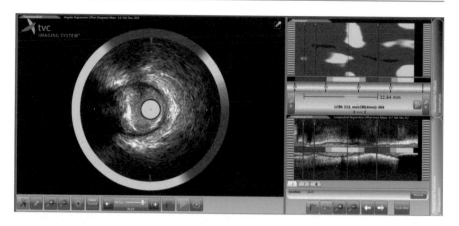

Fig. 9.7 TVC Composite™ view of co-registered near-infrared spectroscopy lipid core plaque with intravascular ultrasound. The chemogram displays low probability of lipid as red and high probability as yellow. The lipid core burden index (LCBI) indicates the amount of lipid in the scanned artery on a 0–1,000 scale

of scattering and absorption of near-infrared light by organic molecules in the arterial wall and plaque produces a unique chemical signature. Then, an algorithm analyzes the detected signal for signs of cholesterol and provide automated LCP detection without the need for manual image processing (Fig. 9.7). In contrast to OCT, NIRS can image through blood, as it does not need light to be directly reflected back to the detector [1].

Equipment TVC Insight Catheter

Minimum guide catheter	6 French (2 mm)
Maximum guidewire	0.014 (0.36)
Catheter crossing tip profile	3.2 French (1.1 mm)
Maximum imaging depth	16 mm
Catheter working length	120 mm
Operating frequency	40 MHz

Limitations NIRS–IVUS doesn't allow detection of non-superficial LCPs and LCPs in large vessels (more than 6 mm diameter) cannot visualize neovascularization [2].

NIRS–IVUS numbers to remember Patient with stable coronary artery disease who undergoes PCI of lesions with large lipid core plaques (maxLCBI4 mm $\geq$500 by NIRS) is associated with a 50 % risk of periprocedural MI [9] and a maxLCBI4 mm >400 in the culprit segment is considered significant with STEMI [10].

Table 9.3 Comparison of three intravascular imaging modalities for the detection of coronary lipid core plaque

	VHIVUS	OCT	NIRS–IVUS
Hybrid intravascular imaging	No	No	Yes
Axial resolution, um	200	10	100
Imaging through blood	++	–	++
Need for blood column clearance during image acquisition	No	Yes	No
Imaging through stents	No	Yes	Yes
Imaging through calcium	No	Yes	Yes for NIRS, no for IVUS
Imaging neovascularization	No	Yes	No
Detection of non-superficial LCPs	Yes	No	No
Evaluation of LCP cap thickness	+	++	*
Detection of thrombus	–	+	*
Expansive remodeling	++	–	++
Need for manual image processing for LCP detection	Yes	Yes	No

++ excellent, + good, – impossible, * potential under investigation, *VHIVUS* virtual histology intravascular ultrasound, *OCT* optical coherence tomography, *NIRS* near-infrared spectroscopy, *LCP* lipid core plaque

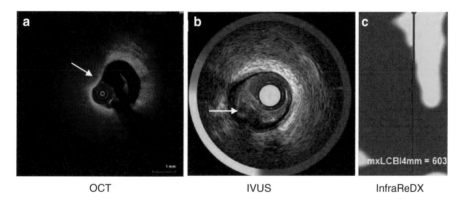

Fig. 9.8 OCT image of a thin-cap fibroatheroma (TCFA) lesion with a 60 μm fibrous cap (*arrow*) overlying a large lipid core (**a**). The lipid pool (*arrow*) is shown in the corresponding IVUS image (**b**). NIRS chemogram quantifies the lipid content of the lesion (**c**)

Multimodality imaging: correlation of OCT and NIRS–IVUS imaging Combined utilization of OCT and NIRS–IVUS allows to characterize the microstructural features of plaque morphology, such as fibrous cap thickness and neovascularization (OCT) and plaque lipid content (NIRS), and perform robust quantitative measurements of lumen, vessel, and plaque area (grayscale IVUS) in the same lesion (Table 9.3). Figure 9.8 shows an example of multimodality images of a thin-cap fibroatheroma lesion.

References

1. Vlodaver Z, Frech R, Van Tassel RA, Edwards JE. Correlation of the antemortem coronary arteriogram and the postmortem specimen. Circulation. 1973;47:162–9.
2. Zir LM, Miller SW, Dinsmore RE, Gilbert JP, Harthorne JW. Interobserver variability in coronary angiography. Circulation. 1976;53:627–32.
3. Gaster AL, Slothuus Skjoldborg U, Larsen J, et al. Continued improvement of clinical outcome and cost effectiveness following intravascular ultrasound guided PCI: insights from a prospective, randomised study. Heart. 2003;89:1043–9.
4. Fitzgerald PJ, Oshima A, Hayase M, et al. Final results of the Can Routine Ultrasound Influence Stent Expansion (CRUISE) study. Circulation. 2000;102:523–30.
5. Koo BK, Yang HM, Doh JH, et al. Optimal intravascular ultrasound criteria and their accuracy for defining the functional significance of intermediate coronary stenoses of different locations. JACC Cardiovasc Interv. 2011;4:803–11.
6. Kang SJ, Lee JY, Ahn JM, et al. Validation of intravascular ultrasound-derived parameters with fractional flow reserve for assessment of coronary stenosis severity. Circ Cardiovasc Interv. 2011;4:65–71.
7. McCabe JM, Croce KJ. Optical CoherenceTomography. Circulation. 2012;126(17):2140.
8. Prati F, Di Vito L, Biondi-Zoccai G, et al. Angiography alone versus angiography plus optical coherence tomography to guide decision-making during percutaneous coronary intervention: the Centro per la Lotta contro l'Infarto-Optimisation of Percutaneous Coronary Intervention (CLI-OPCI) study. EuroIntervention. 2012;8:823–9.
9. Goldstein JA, Maini B, et al. Detection of lipid-core plaques by intracoronary near-infrared spectroscopy identifies high risk of periprocedural myocardial infarction. Circ Cardiovasc Interv. 2011;4(5):429–37.
10. Madder RD, Goldstein JA, et al. Detection by near-infrared spectroscopy of large lipid core plaques at culprit sites in patients with acute ST-segment elevation myocardial infarction. JACC Cardiovasc Interv. 2013;6(8):838–46.

Basics of Intracoronary Devices

10

Ravinder Singh Rao, Anitha Rajamanickam,
and Annapoorna Kini

In the present era of interventional cardiology, with the introduction of newer and more advanced devices on a yearly basis there are various intracoronary devices apart from stents and balloon which have found their place in the catheterization laboratory. This chapter outlines basic coronary devices and their usage.

Balloons

1. Compliant/semi-compliant balloons
2. Noncompliant balloons
3. Cutting balloon (Flextome™)
4. Scoring balloon (AngioSculpt™)
5. Over the wire balloons

Presently, the rapid exchange coronary balloon is used for routine coronary intervention.

Compliant Balloon

- Used for predilation, opening the stent struts, and CTO dilatation
- Advantage: better crossing profile than noncompliant balloon

R.S. Rao, MD • A. Kini, MD, MRCP, FACC (✉) • A. Rajamanickam, MD
Department of Interventional Cardiology, Mount Sinai Hospital,
One Gustave Levy Place, Madison Avenue, New York 10029, NY, USA
e-mail: drravindersinghrao@yahoo.co.in; Annapoorna.kini@mountsinai.org;
Anitha.rajamanickam@mountsinai.org

© Springer-Verlag London 2014
A. Kini et al. (eds.), *Practical Manual of Interventional Cardiology*,
DOI 10.1007/978-1-4471-6581-1_10

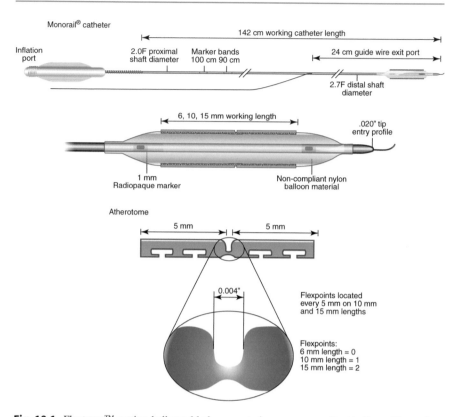

Fig. 10.1 Flextome™ cutting balloon: blades mounted on a noncompliant balloon. Flex points are located every 5 mm on the balloon (Being redrawn by illustrators. ©2014 Boston Scientific Corporation or its affiliates. All rights reserved (Used with permission of Boston Scientific Corporation))

Noncompliant Balloon

- Used for postdilation and predilation of a calcified lesion with or without atherectomy (balloon should be 1:1 to vessel diameter in order to achieve complete expansion)
- Advantage: high-pressure lesion or stent dilatation with little change in balloon reference diameter.

Cutting Balloon (Flextome™)

- Noncompliant balloon
- Blade or atherotome over its surface which cuts the plaque (Fig. 10.1)
- Prevents vessel recoil

- Uses:
  - Calcified lesions
  - Ostial lesions
  - Bifurcation lesions
  - In-stent restenosis
- How to use?
  - Sizing of Flextome™: For native 1:1 sizing and upper inflation limit is 8 atm. For ISR lesion size a quarter size more than the reference vessel. Flextome at 8–10 atm can be used.
  - Rapid exchange or over the wire system.
  - Two cuts are made. Balloon is deflated and pulled into the guide after first inflation and then readvanced for the second cut/inflation.

Scoring Balloon (AngioSculpt™)

- High-pressure balloon with nitinol wire wrapped around, which anchors the balloon to the lesion.
- Use is similar to Flextome, but higher pressure (upto 22 atm) can be achieved with AngioSculpt™.

Coronary Stents

Coronary stent is a mesh of metal or bioabsorbable polymer, non-coated or coated with antiproliferative drug, which is delivered inside the coronary to treat stenotic lesions.

Classification

- Bare metal stents
- Drug-eluting stents
  - First generation: Cypher™, Taxus™
  - Second–third generation: Xience™, Promus™, and Resolute™
- Bioabsorbable Stents

Components of Stent

- Metal Mesh:
  - Design: open cell/closed cell
  - Tensile strength of stent
  - Radial strength
  - Longitudinal foreshortening
- Polymer:
  - Carries the drug.
  - Determines drug kinetics. Duration of drug release affects the restenosis rate.
- Drug:
  - Inhibits cell proliferation thereby preventing restenosis

GuideLiner

Support catheter designed on the basis of "mother–daughter" concept (Fig. 10.2)

Components

- Distal rapid exchange 25 cm extension segment:
  - Inner PTFE coated
  - Middle stainless steel braid to provide support
  - Outer polymer-coated material to provide lubricity and prevent ostial damage
- Collar: proximal end of rapid exchange segment (away from tip)
- 125 cm stainless steel push rod
- Sizes: 5.5F, 6F, 7F

Use

- Deep seating of guide (Fig. 10.3)
- For extra backup support
- Distal delivery of devices
- For coaxial alignment

Technical Tips

- Flush the device from the tip.
- Select the device appropriate to guide.
- Advance over a wire into the guide.
- Advance a balloon into the coronary.
- Advance the GuideLiner over the balloon shaft deep into the vessel. This technique prevents GuideLiner-induced dissection.
- Length of GuideLiner inside the coronary is directly proportional to the amount of support.

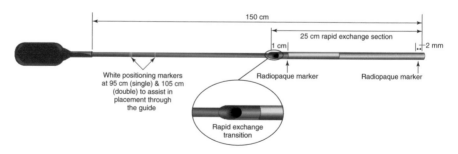

Fig. 10.2 GuideLiner: "guide extension" provides support for complex interventions (Being redrawn by illustrators)

Fig. 10.3 GuideLiner: "mother and child" GuideLiner extending beyond guide catheter into the coronary (Being redrawn by illustrators)

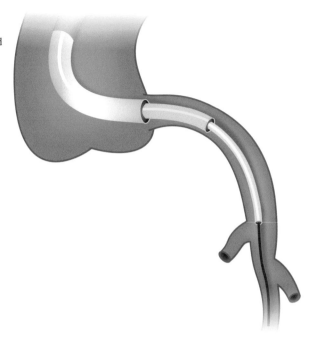

- Do not inject contrast with GuideLiner deep into the coronary, especially when the pressure is damped.
- Exchange the balloon for a stent after appropriate predilation.

Heartrail Catheter

- Based on "mother–daughter" concept of guide extension.
- 125 cm guide passed through a 100 cm guide. No rapid exchange.
- Soft atraumatic tip prevents vessel damage during deep intubation.
- PTFE-coated inner layer, stainless steel braid in middle layer. The largest inner diameter allowing kissing balloon inflation.
- Advance over a wire or PTCA balloon into the distal segment.
- Mainly used for CTO intervention.

Thrombus Aspiration Catheter

Types

- Mechanical:
    - AngioJet™: 4F and 5F.
    - X-Sizer™: Cut and aspirate device. Not FDA approved.

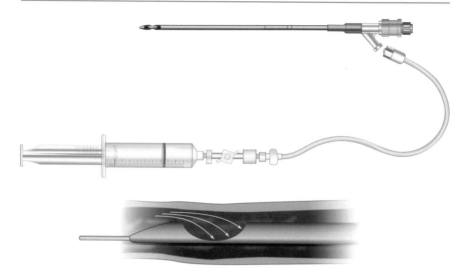

Fig. 10.4 Thrombus aspiration catheter 30 ml locking aspiration syringe. Two-way stopcock. Y-connector. Yellow hub is the stylet

- Manual:
  - Export™: 6F, 7F
  - Pronto Device™
  - Diver CE™
  - Fetch Catheter™

Mechanism

- Rapid exchange/over the wire system.
- Mechanical devices pulverize the thrombus with a jet of saline and aspirate through other ports by the mechanism of Venturi–Bernouli effect.
- Manual device aspirate by negative suction with a 30 cc locking syringe.

Pronto™ (Fig. 10.4 and Table 10.1)

- Kink resistant.
- Distal 18 cm hydrophilic coating.
- Unique distal tip:
  - Tapered entry: protect distal vessel and navigation
  - Self-centering: prevents vessel adhesion while thrombus extraction
  - Sloped extraction lumen: to aspirate large thrombus
- Aspiration syringe is connected to the back end of manual aspiration device and then locked at the stopcock at the hub the syringe piston is pulled negatively and locked, thereby creating a negative pressure inside the syringe.
- The device is advanced distal to the thrombus.
- On opening the stopcock at the hub, blood and thrombus is sucked back into the syringe.
- The catheter is pulled back in a steady and slow motion. Multiple runs are performed as required.

Table 10.1 Sizes of Pronto™

Size	Guide compatibility	Sheath compatibility[a]	Guidewire	Minimum vessel size	Working length
5.5F	6F	5F	0.0014	1.75 mm	138 cm
6.0F	6F	5F	0.0014	2.00 mm	138 cm
7.0F	7F	6F	0.0014	2.25 mm	138 cm
8.0F	8F	7F	0.0014	2.50 mm	138 cm
Pronto LP[b]					
4.0F	6F	6F	0.0014	1.5 mm	140 cm

[a]For peripheral use where guide catheter is not used
[b]Preloaded with a stylet in a lumen different from aspiration to provide kink resistance and push-ability. Rapid exchange length of 20 cm. Most commonly used in coronary interventions

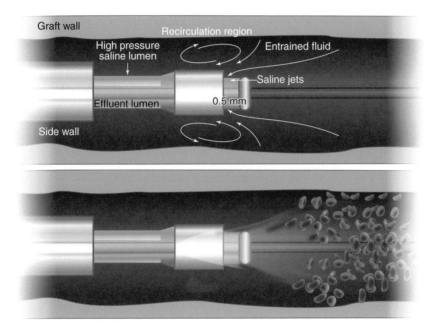

Fig. 10.5 AngioJet catheter. Separate lumen for saline injection and for aspiration creating a low-pressure area (Being redrawn by illustrators)

- After the catheter is removed, the back end of the guide is opened and a generous amount of bleed back is allowed.
- Minimum of 2–3 runs are required.
- The syringe and catheter aspirate is then examined for any thrombus.

AngioJet™

- Select the device (Fig. 10.5):
  - 4F AngioJet™ requires 6F guide.
  - 5F AngioJet™ is useful in vessels >5 mm and SVG interventions and needs 7F guide.

- Prime outside the body by dipping in saline.
- Advance till the proximal part of lesion.
- AngioJet™ is switched to aspirate from proximal to distal.
- Disadvantages:
  - Difficult to deliver in tortuous vessels, distal segment, and calcified vessels
  - Dissection
  - Migration of thrombus
  - Stent deformation (proximal) if attempt is made to pass beyond the stent
- Use:
  - STEMI in setting of primary PCI
  - Vein graft intervention with large thrombus
  - Coronary ectasia/aneurysm with thrombus and requiring intervention
  - For drug delivery in distal vessel

Rotational/Orbital Atherectomy

See Chap. 22

Covered Stents: JOSTENT GraftMaster

- Two stainless steel stents and in between expandable PTFE material (Fig. 10.6)
- Over the wire system and rapid exchange system
- Approved by FDA as a humanitarian device
- Sizes: 2.8, 3, 3.5, 4, 4.5, and 4.8 mm in 13, 18, 23, and 27 mm length
- Use:
  - Coronary perforation
  - Coronary aneurysm requiring treatment
  - Coronary artery fistula requiring treatment
- Technical tips:
  - Preferable guide 7F.
  - 6F guide can be used for 2.8 to less than 4.5 mm stents.

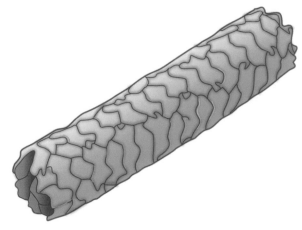

Fig. 10.6 PTFE mesh in between two laser cut stainless steel (Being redrawn by illustrators)

- Rewire with extra support wire like Mailman or Iron Man.
- 300 cm PTCA wire for OTW system.
- Can be used for vessels ≥2.5 cm.
- Anticipate difficulty in delivery.
- Side branch closure if present at the site of rupture.
- Difficult delivery into distal or tortuous or calcified vessels.
- Higher incidence of ISR and thrombosis.

Embolic Protection Devices (EPD) (Fig. 10.7)

Types

Distal Occlusion Devices

- PercuSurge GuardWire
- TriActive system

Proximal Protection Devices

- Mainly used for carotid interventions.
- Prototype: Parodi system, MOMA device

PercuSurge GuardWire

- 0.014 nitinol distal wire (guard wire)
- Occlusion balloon 3.5 cm proximal to terminal end of wire
- Steps:
  - Balloon is inflated to 2–5 atm depending on vessel size.
  - Stent is deployed over the guard wire.
  - Material is aspirated using an Export or Pronto catheter (2–3 runs).
  - Distal balloon is then deflated.
- Advantages:
  - Low crossing profile (0.026–0.033)
  - Traps small and large particles and soluble particles
- Limitations:
  - Complete occlusion of antegrade flow.
  - Single guidewire
  - Collection of material in fornices of balloon

Distal Filter Devices

- Prototypes:
  - FilterWire EZ
  - SpiderFX
- Advantages:
  - Maintains distal perfusion while trapping particles >100 μm

Distal occlusion

Distal filters

Proximal occlusion/
flow reversal

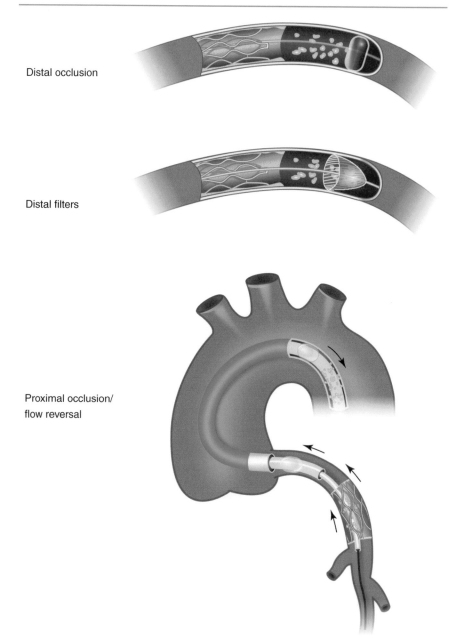

Fig. 10.7 Embolic protection devices: (**a**) distal occlusion balloon. Debris is aspirated before deflating the balloon. (**b**) Filter which traps the embolic debris. Filter is retrieved post procedure by ensheathing it carefully so as not to embolize from the filter: partial capture or complete capture. (**c**) Proximal occlusion device. Useful when distal landing zone is not present. Mainly used for carotid interventions. Balloon is occluded proximal to the lesion and flow is reversed post procedure (Being redrawn by illustrators)

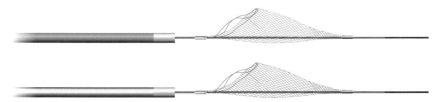

Fig. 10.8 Spider filter: ensheath the filter after stabilizing at the desired position (Being redrawn by illustrators)

- Disadvantages:
    - High crossing profile (0.04–0.05) of sheaths required to keep devices in their collapsed state.
    - Difficulty in crossing the stenosis.
    - Difficulty in advancing retrieval catheter across the stented segment.

Spider Filter

- Sizes: 3–7 mm. Select size 1 mm greater than the vessel diameter (Fig. 10.8).
- 320/190 cm snap wire which moves independent of filter longitudinally.
- Nitinol mesh for complete vessel apposition.
- Steps:
    - Deployed and retrieved through a dual-ended catheter.
    - Compatible with 6F guide and 0.014–0.018 wire.
    - Crossing profile 3.2F.
    - Flush from the distal end.
    - Filter is withdrawn inside the sheath (transparent part in mid segment of sheath) by ensuring that it is immersed in saline the whole time.
    - Advanced as a monorail over the wire which was used to cross the lesion. Park it in a normal segment well beyond the lesion.
    - PTCA wire is removed. The sheath is removed thereby deploying the filter.
    - Filter after completion of the intervention, the filter is retrieved by sheathing the device and removing the whole system.

FilterWire EZ System™

- Components:
    - Wire
    - Delivery sheath
    - Retrieval sheath
    - Torquer, peel-away introducer, and valve dilator
- Sizes:
    - Two sizes for the following range of coronary artery sizes with wire length of 190 or 300 cm [2.25–3.5 and 3.5–5.5 mm].

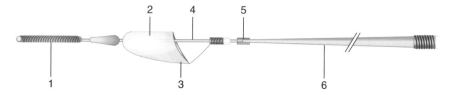

Fig. 10.9 (*1*) Radiopaque tip (2 and 3 cm for two systems, respectively). (*2*) Filter. (*3*) Radiopaque nitinol loop. (*4*) Spinner tube. (*5*) Proximal loop. (*6*) PTFE-coated wire (0.014) (Being redrawn by illustrators)

- Landing zone:
    - Landing zone is the distance from distal edge of lesion to tip of radiopaque part (Fig. 10.9). It is the normal segment of the vessel where filter can be deployed.
        - For 2.25–3.5 mm system: ≥2.5 mm
        - For 3.5–5.5 mm system: ≥3 mm

Intravascular Brachytherapy (IVBT)

- Indication: to reduce the recurrence of in-stent restenosis
- Mechanism: locally applied radiation can block or attenuate local tissue proliferation causing ISR
- Effects of brachytherapy:
    - Delayed recurrent restenosis
    - Late stent thrombosis because of prolonged inhibition of intimal formation
    - Late vessel stent separation because of positive remodeling
    - Geographical miss: reactive hyperproliferation at the edges because of less radiation dose
- Types of brachytherapy: both gamma and beta sources are effective, but only beta source is clinically available.
- Properties of beta radiation:
    - Low energy
    - Less shielding
    - Shorter delivery time
- *FDA-approved brachytherapy systems:*
    - Gamma: Cordis Checkmate™
    - Beta: Novoste Beta-Cath™ and Guidant Galileo™

Novoste Beta-Cath™

- Clinically used in the USA
- Guide selection: 6Fr
- Wire: 0.014
- Distal 1 cm rapid exchange length

- Selection of device and steps:
  - Based on the length of the injury:
    - Treated with 20 mm balloon for a 30 or 40 mm system
    - Injury area up to 40 mm for 60 mm system
  - Diameter of the reference vessel should be between 2.7 and 4 mm.
  - Balloon predilation of ISR is done.
  - No stent is placed when IVBT is planned because of increased risk of stent thrombosis.
  - Dual antiplatelet is continued lifelong.
  - In long lesion serial delivery of catheter with 1 mm overlap is recommended. We recommend adequate anticoagulation with bivalurudin (to an ACT of >300) and an additional dose of 2500 units of heparin IV just before delivery of the radiation dose.

BridgePoint System™ (CTO Devices)

Components

- CorssBoss™: blunt-tipped catheter to pass the occlusion and for subintimal entry
- Stingray™: flat-shaped balloon with side exit holes (Fig. 10.10)
- Guidewire: a small-diameter wire with an angled and sharpened tip for reentry into true lumen

Inflate Stingray balloon up to 4 atm in subintimal space, and attempt reentry into true lumen with guidewire.

Corsair Catheter™

- Hydrophilic-coated distal 60 cm (Fig. 10.11).
- Tungsten braiding +10 elliptical stainless steel braids.
- Outer diameter is 2.8F and tapers to 0.016 in.
- Length is 135 cm for antegrade and 150 cm for retrograde.
- Characteristics:
  - Excellent pushability, flexibility, and torqueability
  - Kink-resistant tip
  - Helpful in crossing microchannels in CTO
  - Used for retrograde CTO PCI
  - Provides support to guidewire and useful for guidewire exchange

Twin-Pass Catheter

- Double-lumen exchange catheter (Fig. 10.12)
- One rapid exchange lumen and one over the wire

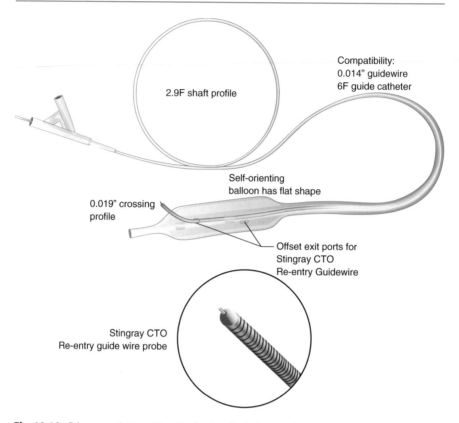

Fig. 10.10 Stingray catheter with self-orienting flat balloon and a reentry port (Being redrawn by illustrators)

- Hydrophilic coating present
- Length: 140 cm
- 3Fr system
- Guide compatibility: ≥5F for 0.014 system which is most commonly used for coronary intervention
- Use:
  - Flush both lumens prior to use.
  - To deliver drugs distally into coronary circulation.
  - To image distally with contrast.
  - To exchange wire while keeping one wire in place.

Catheters for Difficult Wiring of Side Branches or Angulated Lesions

Venture Catheter

- Over the wire system or monorail (Fig. 10.13).
- Deflectable tip, which can be controlled by rotating a knob on the device.

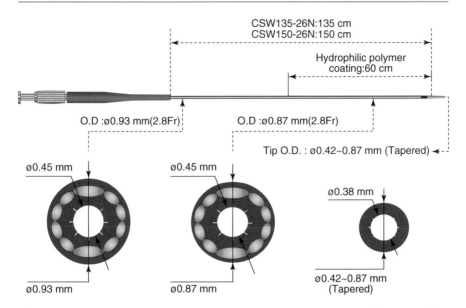

Fig. 10.11 Images of Corsair microcatheter illustrating tapered tip and hydrophilic nature (Being redrawn by illustrators)

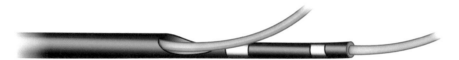

Fig. 10.12 Twin-pass catheter. The second lumen (over the wire) can be used for the second wire or delivering of contrast or drug distally (Being redrawn by illustrators)

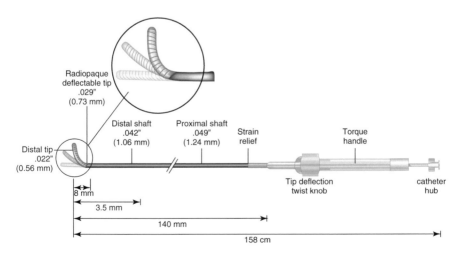

Fig. 10.13 Venture catheter: deflectable tip which helps in directing the wire in angulated side branches. Tip can be deflected by rotating the knob (Being redrawn by illustrators)

Fig. 10.14 SuperCross catheter: preshaped microcatheter to wire angulated side branches (Being redrawn by illustrators)

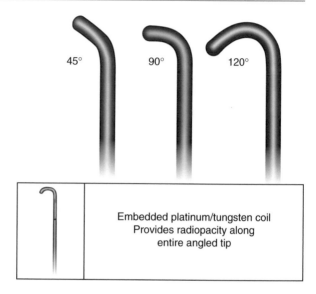

45° 90° 120°

Embedded platinum/tungsten coil
Provides radiopacity along
entire angled tip

- How to use?
  - Advance the wire beyond the origin of side branch into the main vessel.
  - Advance Venture catheter over the wire beyond the side branch to be entered.
  - Pull back the wire inside Venture.
  - Rotate the knob so as to orient the tip of Venture catheter to the angle of side branch origin.
  - Pull back the catheter till the ostium of side branch.
  - Once the Venture is at the origin of side branch, advance the wire.
- Complications:
  - Dissection of the main vessel
  - Dissection of side branch

SuperCross Catheter

- Has prefixed tip angles. The most commonly used angles are 90° and 120° (Fig. 10.14).
- Rapid exchange system.
- Selected depending on the angle of side branch.
- How to use?
  - Advance the wire beyond the side branch origin in main vessel.
  - Advance the SuperCross catheter on the wire, beyond side branch.
  - Pull back the wire and the tip of SuperCross will assume its preshaped angle.
  - Pull back the SuperCross and orient it to the origin of side branch.
  - Advance the wire into side branch.
- Complications:
  - Dissection of main vessel
  - Dissection of side branch

Hemodynamic Assessment: Right Heart Catheterization, Pulmonary Hypertension, Left-to-Right Shunt, and Constriction

11

Rikesh Patel, Anitha Rajamanickam, and Ajith Nair

Hemodynamic assessment is a critical function of cardiac catheterization labs. Though significant advances in imaging modalities have replaced many of the functions of hemodynamic assessment, the catheterization laboratory still remains important for accurate measurements and the confirmation of diagnoses, especially in patients with suboptimal or equivocal imaging results

Indications

- Evaluate and perform hemodynamic assessment of valvular heart disease
- Evaluate and confirm the diagnosis of pulmonary hypertension
- Evaluate left-to-right shunt
- Differentiate constrictive from restrictive physiology
- Evaluate complex congenital heart disease (outside the scope of this text)

Contraindications

- Vegetation, tumor or thrombus in the right heart, mechanical prosthesis in the tricuspid or pulmonary position, hemodynamic or electrical instability [1]

Equipment

- 7–8 Fr sheath access kit
- Multi-lumen pulmonary artery (PA) catheter (alternatively, wedge catheter with 5–6 Fr sheath)

R. Patel, MD (✉) • A. Rajamanickam, MD • A. Nair, MD
Department of Interventional Cardiology, Mount Sinai Hospital,
One Gustave Levy Place, Madison Avenue, New York 10029, NY, USA
e-mail: rikeshrpatel@gmail.com, rikeshpatel.md@gmail.com;
Anitha.Rajamanickam@mountsinai.org; Ajith.nair@mountsinai.org

© Springer-Verlag London 2014
A. Kini et al. (eds.), *Practical Manual of Interventional Cardiology*,
DOI 10.1007/978-1-4471-6581-1_11

Access 7–8 Fr femoral, internal jugular vein; 5–7 Fr antecubital (medial preferred)

Fluoroscopic Views Straight anterior-posterior (AP)

Steps for Standard Right Heart Catheterization

- Insert the PA catheter into the sheath (May use a leading J-tipped wire 0.035″, 0.018″ Platinum Plus or Swan wire, or 0.014″ support wire (Grand Slam or Iron Man) if using antecubital approach if needed). Advance the PA catheter to its 20 cm marker and inflate the balloon.
- Float the PA catheter into the right atrium (RA). Flush the system and zero the pressure transducer. Record the RA pressure. Advance the catheter into the right ventricle (RV). After recording the pressure, turn the catheter clockwise, transmitting torque by small back-forth motion of the catheter. When the tip of the catheter faces up in the right ventricular outflow tract (RVOT), advance the catheter (by pushing) into the pulmonary artery. Deep inspiration can assist in floating the catheter into the pulmonary artery. If difficulty is encountered, the catheter can be directed toward the lateral wall of the RA and looped to advance it into the RVOT and PA. If difficulty in floating the catheter persists, a Swan or 0.018″ Platinum Plus wire can be used to guide the catheter into the PA. The balloon should be deflated to allow for easy tracking of the catheter along the support wire. An appropriate pulmonary capillary wedge pressure (PCWP) tracing should be recorded with appropriate transition to PA waveform when the balloon is deflated. If the PCWP is hybridized, attempt advancing the catheter to wedge position with the balloon partially inflated or pull back by a different wedge position. Ideally, all pressure measurements are made at end-expiration (except in ventilated patients).
    - Note, for antecubital approach, it is easiest to allow the leading wire to guide the catheter directly into the PA and measure pressures on catheter pullback.
- For routine, right heart catheterization, measure the PA oxygen saturation. For Fick estimation of cardiac output (CO), arterial oxygen saturation can be assumed from pulse oximetry or measured directly if arterial access is present. Calculate the cardiac output and index by the Fick method (oxygen consumption is assumed, but can be measured directly).
- If using a PA catheter, connect the cable for thermodilution measurement of cardiac output and firmly inject 10 cc of saline in the proximal port (repeat two to three times). Thermodilution method may be omitted if severe tricuspid/pulmonic regurgitation is present.
- If severe pulmonary hypertension is present, and unexplained by pulmonary venous hypertension (normal PCWP), consider vasoreactivity testing (see below).
- If PA saturation is >75 % on repeated measurement and is not otherwise well explained (high-output state), an oxygen saturation run should be performed for detection and quantification of left-to-right shunt (see below).

Steps for Evaluation of Pulmonary Hypertension

- Perform standard right heart catheterization as described above. Calculate the transpulmonary gradient (TPG) and pulmonary vascular resistance (PVR). If there is doubt regarding the accuracy of the wedge pressure, a simultaneous left ventricular end-diastolic pressure should be measured via left heart catheterization.

$$\text{Transpulmonary gradient}\,(\text{TPG}) = \text{Mean PAP} - \text{PCWP}$$
$$\text{PVR}\,(\text{Woods}) = \text{TPG}\,(\text{mmHg}) / \text{CO}\,(\text{L} / \text{min})$$

- If pulmonary arterial hypertension is present, defined by mean PA pressure >25 mmHg and a PVR >3 Wood units, and PCWP (and/or LVEDP) <15 mmHg, then acute vasodilator testing should be performed [2].
- For vasoreactivity testing, we administer inhaled nitric oxide at a dose of 40 parts per million (ppm) for 5 min, with continuous hemodynamic monitoring [3, 4]. Responders (or reactivity) to vasodilator testing (for purposes of initiating calcium channel blocker therapy) are defined as demonstrating a decrease in mean PAP by 10 mmHg to a mean PAP less than 40 mmHg without a decrease in cardiac output [2].

Steps for Evaluation of Left-to-Right Shunt

- Perform standard right heart catheterization as described above. Oxygen saturations can be measured on advancement or pullback of the catheter. When left-to-right shunt is not clinically suspected, a screening PA oxygen saturation should be measured; if the value is >75 % and unexplained by high cardiac output state and/or AV fistula, a complete saturation run should be performed.
- Oxygen saturations should be obtained from the pulmonary artery, right ventricle, right atrium, and superior vena cava. A difference between two chambers of approximately 5–7 % [5] is considered significant.
- Calculation of shunt fraction:
  - Use the difference in oxygen saturation to estimate ratio of flow across pulmonic (Q_p) and systemic circulatory (Q_s) beds:

$$Q_p / Q_s = \frac{\text{Arterial} - \text{Mixed venous}}{\text{Pulmonary venous} - \text{Pulmonary artery}}$$

  - With a few exceptions, arterial saturation can be used as a surrogate for the pulmonary venous saturation.
  - Mixed venous saturation is calculated as (3 SVC saturations +1 IVC saturation)/4 otherwise it is assumed to be equivalent to the saturation from the chamber proximal to the suspected defect (saturation before "step up") and the IVC saturation can generally be excluded due to variability in measurement related to streaming and relative contribution to the average mixed venous saturation.
  - *Exceptions* to use of SVC saturation for mixed venous saturation measurement:
    - Anomalous pulmonary venous return above the SVC/RA junction.

- Arteriovenous fistula or malformation above the SVC/RA junction.
- In general these pitfalls can be overcome by measurement of venous saturation proximal to (above the level of) the shunts, if possible.
- Shunt calculation is not reliable in patent ductus arteriosus due to the distal site of shunting.

Complications While complications are generally rare (<1 %), the most common complications are access related (hematoma, pneumothorax). Additional adverse events may include usually transient arrhythmia due to catheter stimulation, vagal-induced hypotension, or reactions to vasoreactivity testing [6]. Vasoreactivity testing should be generally avoided in patients with significant, decompensated left heart disease or venoocclusive disease due to risk of pulmonary edema [2].

Post-procedural Care manual compression for hemostasis and routine post-procedural monitoring of vital signs

Steps for Evaluation of Constriction Versus Restriction

- Perform standard right heart catheterization as described above.
- Perform standard left heart catheterization, ideally with a pigtail catheter in the left ventricle.
- After zeroing both transducers and documenting simultaneous PCWP/LVEDP, deflate the PA catheter balloon and withdraw it slowly, until it falls into the right ventricle. The balloon can be reinflated in the RV to reduce ectopy.
- Slow the sweep speed and equalize the scales for measurement of simultaneous LV and RV pressures.
- If RA pressure was <15 mmHg, administer 1 litre of normal saline (fluid challenge).
- Hemodynamic tracings of LV/RV pressures typically demonstrate a "dip and plateau" or "square root sign" and, in constriction, usually with equalization of diastolic pressures.
- Hemodynamic criteria suggestive of constriction are included in Table 11.1:

Table 11.1 Hemodynamic criteria suggestive of constriction

	Constriction	Restriction
LVEDP–RVEDP (mmHg)	≤5	>5
PASP (mmHg)	≤55	>55
RVEDP/RVSP	>1/3	<1/3
Inspiratory fall in RAP (mmHg)	<5	>5
Inspiratory decrease in PCWP>LVDP	Present	Absent
Systolic area index	>1.1	<1.1

- In *constriction*, during inspiration, there is an *increase in the area of the RV* pressure curve (compared with expiration), and due to interventricular dependence, there is a simultaneous *decrease in the area of the LV* pressure curve.

$$\text{The systolic area index} = \frac{[RV\,area\,/\,LV\,area]_{inspiration}}{[RV\,area\,/\,LV\,area]_{expiration}}$$

  - Systolic area index >1.1 is highly suggestive of constriction [7].

References

1. Mueller HS, et al. ACC expert consensus document. Present use of bedside right heart catheterization in patients with cardiac disease. J Am Coll Cardiol. 1998;32(3):840–64.
2. McLaughlin VV, et al. ACCF/AHA 2009 expert consensus document on pulmonary hypertension a report of the American College of Cardiology Foundation Task Force on Expert Consensus Documents and the American Heart Association developed in collaboration with the American College of Chest Physicians; American Thoracic Society, Inc.; and the Pulmonary Hypertension Association. J Am Coll Cardiol. 2009;53(17):1573–619.
3. Pepke-Zaba J, et al. Inhaled nitric oxide as a cause of selective pulmonary vasodilatation in pulmonary hypertension. Lancet. 1991;338(8776):1173–4.
4. Krasuski RA, et al. Inhaled nitric oxide selectively dilates pulmonary vasculature in adult patients with pulmonary hypertension, irrespective of etiology. J Am Coll Cardiol. 2000;36(7):2204–11.
5. Baim DS, Grossman W. Grossman's cardiac catheterization, angiography, and intervention. 7th ed. Philadelphia: Lippincott Williams & Wilkins; 2006. xvii, 807 p.
6. Hoeper MM, et al. Complications of right heart catheterization procedures in patients with pulmonary hypertension in experienced centers. J Am Coll Cardiol. 2006;48(12):2546–52.
7. Talreja DR, et al. Constrictive pericarditis in the modern era: novel criteria for diagnosis in the cardiac catheterization laboratory. J Am Coll Cardiol. 2008;51(3):315–9.

Hemodynamic Assessment of Aortic/ Mitral Stenosis and Regurgitation

12

Rikesh Patel, Anitha Rajamanickam, and Annapoorna Kini

Aortic Stenosis

Indications Evaluation of aortic stenosis of uncertain severity and/or in preparation for balloon aortic valvuloplasty and surgical or transcatheter aortic valve replacement

Contraindications Mechanical aortic valve, active vegetation, and LV thrombus (see Chap. 11)

Equipment 7.5 and 6 Fr sheaths

- Pulmonary artery catheter or wedge catheter
- 5 Fr AR2 catheter
- Optional: dual-lumen pigtail catheter (Langston)[R]
- Straight-tip Terumo Glidewire™
- Manifolds (3) and transducers

Access 7.5 Fr venous, 6 Fr arterial

Fluoroscopic Views Left anterior oblique [LAO] (for aortography, crossing)

R. Patel, MD (✉) • A. Rajamanickam, MD • A. Kini, MD, MRCP, FACC
Department of Interventional Cardiology, Mount Sinai Hospital,
One Gustave Levy Place, Madison Avenue, New York 10029, NY, USA
e-mail: rikeshrpatel@gmail.com, rikeshpatel.md@gmail.com; arajamanickam@gmail.com,
Anitha.Rajamanickam@mountsinai.org; Annapoorna.kini@mountsinai.org

© Springer-Verlag London 2014
A. Kini et al. (eds.), *Practical Manual of Interventional Cardiology*,
DOI 10.1007/978-1-4471-6581-1_12

Steps

- Perform a right heart catheterization, obtaining right atrial (RA), right ventricular (RV), pulmonary artery (PA), and pulmonary capillary wedge (PCW) pressures, along with PA saturation for calculation of cardiac output (CO), optional measurement of CO by thermodilution method. Leave the PA catheter in the pulmonary artery.
- Assess left coronary anatomy by usual techniques (limited AP caudal/cranial projections for the left coronary system, unless otherwise indicated).
- Connect femoral artery (FA) sheath to pressure. Advance a 5Fr AR2 diagnostic catheter (over a standard 0.035″ J-wire) to the ascending aorta. Flush the catheter and zero all transducers simultaneously. Record simultaneous pressures from the FA sheath and AR2 catheter. If the gradient is >10 mmHg, consider exchanging for a dual-lumen pigtail catheter (Langston) to accurately evaluate the pressure gradient across the aortic valve (after crossing into the LV).
- Perform an aortogram in the (LAO) projection (20–25°) to elucidate the valve orifice, degree of aortic regurgitation, and right coronary artery (RCA) takeoff.
- Engage and perform a single right coronary angiogram (LAO/AP cranial projection, unless otherwise indicated).
- Administer heparin 2,000 units IV/IA.
- In the LAO projection, use the AR2 catheter to direct a straight-tip Terumo Glidewire™ across the aortic valve; upon crossing with the wire, advance the AR2 catheter into the LV over the wire (preferably in the right anterior oblique [RAO] projection).
- Remove the wire, zero all transducers, and assess the LV-FA gradient. If a significant (>10 mmHg) FA-central aortic gradient was previously noted, exchange the AR2 catheter for a dual-lumen pigtail catheter (Langston[R]) over an exchange length 0.035″ J-wire.
- Calculate the aortic valve area (AVA) using the Hakki or Gorlin formula [1, 2].
- *Hakki*:

$$\text{Aortic valve area}\left(cm^2\right) \approx \frac{\text{Cardiac output}\left(1/\min\right)}{\sqrt{\text{Peak to peak gradient}\left(mmHg\right)}}$$

- *Gorlin:*

$$\text{Valve area}\left(cm^2\right) = \frac{\text{Cardiac output}\left(ml/\min\right)}{\text{Heart rate}\left(beats/\min\right) \cdot \text{Systolic ejection period}\left(s\right)} \cdot 44.3 \cdot \sqrt{\text{mean gradient}\left(mmHg\right)}$$

- If the mean LV-aortic gradient (see Fig. 12.1) is less than 40 mmHg and the Left ventricular ejection fraction (LVEF) is <40, consider dobutamine infusion (starting at 5 mcg/kg/min, titrating up to 40 mcg/kg/min). If the mean gradient (see Fig. 12.2) is less than 40 mmHg, the Left ventricular ejection fraction (LVEF) is normal, and the patient is hypertensive, consider a nipride challenge (0.25 mcg/kg/min, titrating

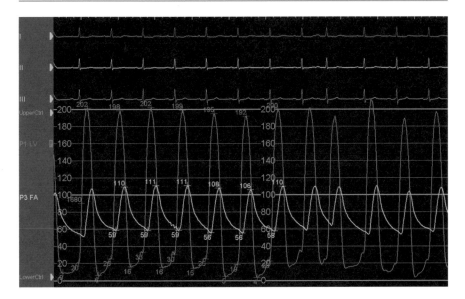

Fig. 12.1 Severe aortic stenosis (LV, aortic pressures)

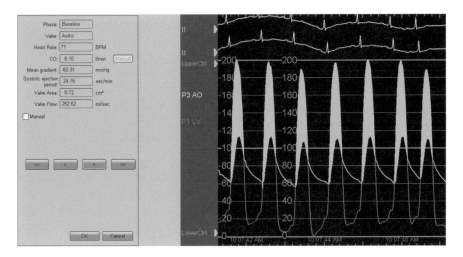

Fig. 12.2 Mean gradient in severe aortic stenosis

up to 10 mcg/kg/min). Repeat hemodynamics, reassessing pressure gradient and cardiac output, and recalculate the valve area. An increase in the valve area suggests more pseudo-stenosis secondary to LV dysfunction. In truly severe AS, the gradient may rise, but the AVA should remain relatively unchanged [3].

• Record simultaneous LV-PCW pressure tracings. If no valvuloplasty is planned, document a pullback to ensure well-matched aortic pressure tracings (regardless of catheter used).

- Severity of AS:
  - Severe: AVA <1 cm^2
  - Moderate: AVA of 1–1.5 cm^2
  - Mild: AVA >1.5 cm^2

Complications Cerebrovascular accident, vascular

Post-procedure Care Routine post-catheterization care

Mitral Stenosis

Indications Evaluation of mitral stenosis severity and/or in preparation for balloon mitral valvuloplasty [4].

Contraindications Mechanical aortic valve, active vegetation, and LV thrombus; contraindications for right heart catheterization (see Chap. 12)

Equipment

- 7.5 Fr and 6 Fr sheaths
- Pulmonary artery catheter or wedge catheter
- Manifolds (3)

Access 7.5 Fr venous, 6 Fr arterial

Fluoroscopic Views AP

Steps

- Perform a right heart catheterization, obtaining right atrial (RA), right ventricular (RV), pulmonary artery (PA), and pulmonary capillary wedge (PCW) pressures, along with PA saturation for calculation of cardiac output (CO), optional measurement of CO by thermodilution method. Leave the PA catheter in the pulmonary artery.
- Advance a 5 Fr pigtail catheter (over a standard 0.035″ J-wire) to the left ventricle. Flush the catheter and zero all transducers simultaneously. Record simultaneous pressures from the LV and PCW positions (see Fig. 12.3) in order to document the transmitral gradient (see Fig. 12.4).
- Calculate the mitral valve area (MVA) using the Hakki (above) or modified Gorlin formula:

$$\text{Mitral valve area} = \frac{\text{Cardiac output}}{\left(\text{Diastolic filling period}\right)\left(\text{Heart rate}\right)\left(37.9\right)\left(\sqrt{\text{Pressure gradient}}\right)}$$

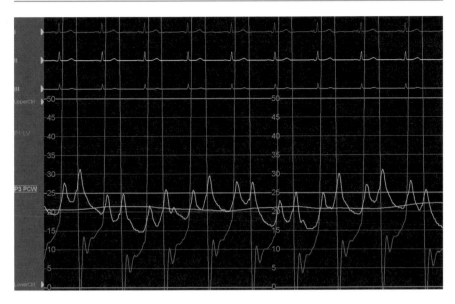

Fig. 12.3 Resting hemodynamics in severe mitral stenosis (LV, PCW pressures)

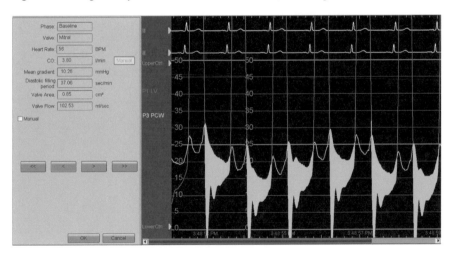

Fig. 12.4 Resting mean gradient in mitral stenosis

- If mild mitral stenosis is present, consider exercise with continuous hemodynamic monitoring to evaluate for an increase in the gradient (>15 mm Hg) and/or a significant rise in pulmonary artery pressure (systolic >60 mmHg) and/or a significant rise is pulmonary capillary wedge pressure (≥25) (Figs. 12.5, 12.6, 12.7, and 12.8).
- Perform a left ventriculogram to evaluate for mitral regurgitation (30 cc volume for 20 cc/s @ 450 PSI, RAO 30–45).
- Perform an aortogram to evaluate for aortic regurgitation (40 cc volume for 20 cc/s @ 650 PSI, LAO 30–45).

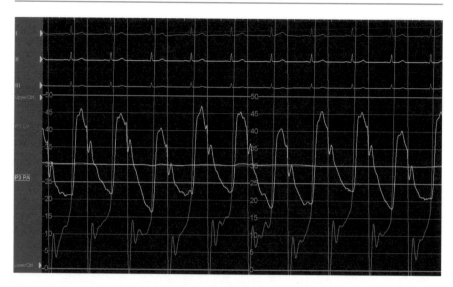

Fig. 12.5 Resting pulmonary artery pressure in severe MS

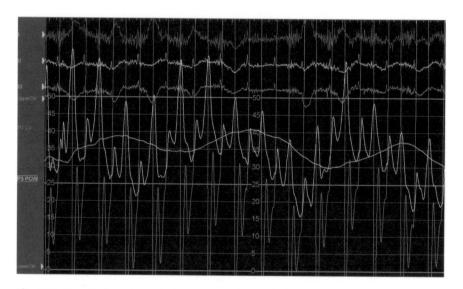

Fig. 12.6 Exercise hemodynamics in severe mitral stenosis (LV, PCWP)

- Engage and perform right and left coronary angiography (unless not indicated).
- Transseptal catheterization and measurement of left atrial pressure is required if the diagnosis is unclear and mechanical aortic valve or LV thrombus is present.

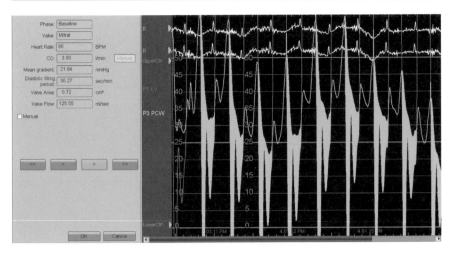

Fig. 12.7   Exercise mean gradient in mitral stenosis

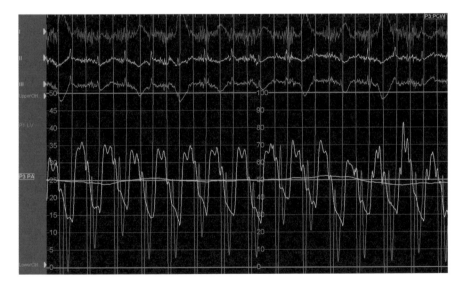

Fig. 12.8   Exercise pulmonary pressures in severe MS

- Intrapulmonary nitroglycerin (200–300 mcg) may be injected to rule out falsely elevated gradient caused by pulmonary venous hypertension.
- Severity of MS:
  - Severe: MVA <1 cm^2
  - Moderate: MVA of 1–1.5 cm^2
  - Mild: MVA >1.5 cm^2

Complications Vascular

Post-procedure Care Routine post-catheterization care

Mitral and Aortic Regurgitation

Indications Evaluation of valvular regurgitation of uncertain severity and/or in preparation for possible surgical/transcatheter repair or replacement

Contraindications Decompensated heart failure (due to volume load) or other usual contraindications to cardiac catheterization

Equipment

- 5 or 6 Fr pigtail catheter
- Power injector for large-volume contrast injection

Access 5 or 6 Fr arterial

Fluoroscopic Views

- Aortogram – LAO 45 (may require adjustment to ensure the left ventricle is adequately visualized)
- Left ventriculogram – RAO 50 (may require adjustment based on course of aorta and size of ventricle/atrium in relationship to the spine)

Steps for Aortography

- Advance a pigtail catheter over a wire in usual fashion to the ascending aorta. Position the pigtail just above the sinotubular junction, so as to avoid contact with the valve.
- Ensure tubing and connections are free of air and are secure.
- The catheter should be held in position to avoid contact with the aortic valve or migration to an inappropriately high position in the ascending aorta.
- Settings for power injection: 40 cc of contrast, 15 cc/s flow, 750 PSI, 0.0 s rise.

Steps for Left Ventriculography

- Advance a pigtail catheter over a wire in usual fashion into the left ventricle, ensuring the wire (and, therefore, catheter) is free in the ventricular cavity and not entangled with the mitral valvular apparatus.
- Ensure tubing and connections are free of air and secure.
- The catheter should be held in position to avoid migration and ectopy or blow-back into the aorta.

- Settings for power injection: 40 cc of contrast, 15 cc/s flow, 650 PSI, 0.2 s rise.
- Upon injection, panning the table may be required (usually pushing the table away from the operator – standing on the patient's right) to visualize regurgitation into particularly dilated atria.

Quantification of Regurgitation (MR or AI)

- *1+* dye regurgitation to contralateral chamber *without* outlining of the chamber.
- *2+* dye regurgitation to contralateral chamber *with* complete outlining of the chamber, but gradual dye clearance.
- *3+* dye regurgitation with progressive opacification of contralateral chamber in 4–6 beats.
- *4+* dye regurgitation with instantaneous opacification of contralateral chamber in <3 beats. In case of mitral regurgitation, there will be opacification of pulmonary veins.

Complications Cerebrovascular accident, vascular

Post-procedure Care Routine post-catheterization care

References

1. Hakki AH et al. A simplified valve formula for the calculation of stenotic cardiac valve areas. Circulation. 1981;63(5):1050–5.
2. Gorlin R, Gorlin SG. Hydraulic formula for calculation of the area of the stenotic mitral valve, other cardiac valves, and central circulatory shunts. I. Am Heart J. 1951;41(1):1–29.
3. Zile MR, Gaasch WH. Heart failure in aortic stenosis – improving diagnosis and treatment. N Engl J Med. 2003;348(18):1735–6.
4. Baim DS, Grossman W. Grossman's cardiac catheterization, angiography, and intervention. 7th ed. Philadelphia: Lippincott Williams & Wilkins; 2006. xvii, 222–33, 257–63, 807 p.

Vascular Closure Devices and Complications

13

Faramarz (Taj) Tehrani, Anitha Rajamanickam, and Robert Pyo

When compared to manual compression, utilization of vascular closure devices (VCDs) in an appropriate patient population has the potential to reduce time to post procedure mobility and thereby improve patient comfort after percutaneous procedures [1–3]. Additionally, reduced time to ambulation is important as more hospitals adopt same-day discharge strategies. However it has not been clearly established if VCDs reduce overall complication rates when compared to manual compression. When utilizing these devices, one must weigh the potential complications associated with these devices against their potential benefits. This chapter will review VCDs commonly used with respect to their specific indications for use, specific contraindications, and safe deployment practices.

Perclose™ (Abbott Vascular, Abbott Park, IL): Suture-Based Device

Indications

- The vascular access site should be in the common femoral artery.
- The common femoral artery should be at least 5 mm in diameter.
- 6–8 F arteriotomy can be closed.
- 8+ arteriotomy can be closed with multiple Perclose™ pre-deployment called Preclose.

F. (Taj) Tehrani, MD • A. Rajamanickam, MD (✉) • R. Pyo, MD
Department of Interventional Cardiology, Mount Sinai Hospital,
One Gustave Levy Place, Madison Avenue, New York 10029, NY, USA
e-mail: tajtehrani@gmail.com; arajamanickam@gmail.com,
Anitha.rajamanickam@mountsinai.org; Robert.pyo@mountsinai.org

© Springer-Verlag London 2014
A. Kini et al. (eds.), *Practical Manual of Interventional Cardiology*,
DOI 10.1007/978-1-4471-6581-1_13

Contraindications

- Common femoral artery luminal diameter less than 5 mm in diameter
- Significant peripheral vascular disease
  - Significant luminal encroachment
  - More than mild fluoroscopically visible calcification

Deployment Steps

- Place a guidewire (0.038 or less) through the procedural sheath and remove the sheath while applying pressure (Fig. 13.1a).
- Backload the device over the guidewire until the guidewire comes out of the device guidewire exit port. Use of a gauze may help to grip the slippery hydrophilic distal portion of the device (Fig. 13.1b). Rail the device over the guidewire until the guidewire exit port is just above the skin line (Fig. 13.1c).
- Pull the guidewire out and continue to advance the device with gentle side to side rotating motion until (usually) brisk pulsatile flow of blood is evident from the marker lumen (Fig. 13.1d). Note that a slow trickle of blood may be seen if the device is incompletely inserted into the vessel. Continue to push the device forward – often a "give" will be felt as the device is fully inserted.
- Position the device at a 45° angle (angle is usually the same angle used for initial needle entry while obtaining access) and deploy the foot by lifting the lever on the body of the device (Fig. 13.1e).
- Gently pull the device back to position the foot against the arterial wall (Figure Inset). Two things will be evident: (a) There will be firm resistance to further pull back and (b) blood flow from the marker lumen will stop (Fig. 13.1f).
- Stabilize the device with your left hand making sure that firm upward traction is maintained on the device, and with the right hand, deploy needles by pushing on the plunger assembly (Fig. 13.1g).
- While continuing to stabilize the device with the left hand, disengage the needles by pulling the plunger assembly back (Fig. 13.1h), and continue to pull the assembly back until the suture is taut (Fig. 13.1i). Loop the suture around the trimming mechanism located on the body of the device to cut it (Fig. 13.1j).
- Return the foot to its original closed position by pushing the lever down, and pull back on the device with a side to side rotating motion until the guidewire port is visible above the skin line. Pull the ends of the rail (long, blue) and lock (shorter, white tip) sutures from the device and secure them with clamps (or wet gauze) and reinsert the guidewire back in through the port (Fig. 13.1k). (PRECLOSE STEPS: The same above steps are used for Preclose. Make sure that the two sutures as secured with adequate slack to the sterile field using a clamp. A second Preclose may be deployed but turn the device clockwise 90° for deployment as compared to the previously deployed Preclose. Then insert the sheath through the guidewire to perform the necessary intervention. At end of the procedure reinsert a long guidewire through the sheath and remove the sheath and perform the following steps to close the arteriotomy site.)

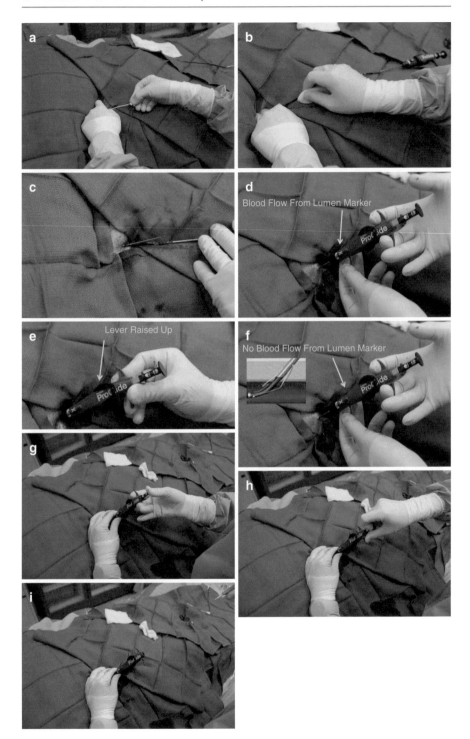

Fig. 13.1 Steps of Perclose closure device deployment

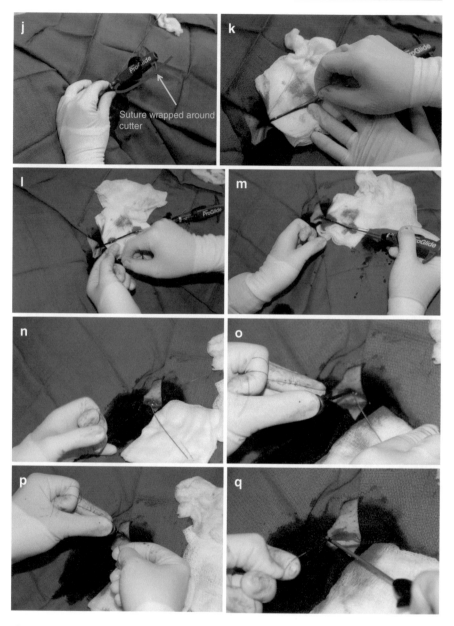

Fig. 13.1 (continued)

- Wrap the rail limb (long, blue) of suture around your left index finger, close to the skin level (Fig. 13.1l).
- Remove the device with the right hand, while maintaining an adequate length of guidewire inside the artery (Fig. 13.1m).

- While removing the device with the right hand, simultaneously advance the knot to the arteriotomy by applying slow, consistent increasing tension to the rail suture limb, keeping the suture coaxial to the tissue tract (Fig. 13.1n).
- If bleeding is controlled, the operator should then remove the guidewire. *If it is evident that hemostasis has not been achieved, the procedure should be aborted at this stage. The suture can be removed by a quick, firm tug on the lock limb of the suture – this will break the knot and allow removal of the entire length of suture. A size 7.5 F (or greater) sheath should be inserted over the wire and manual compression performed when it is safe to do so.*
- Engage the Knot Pusher on the rail limb and push the slip knot to the arteriotomy (Fig. 13.1o). Once the knot is sufficiently pushed down to achieve hemostasis, lock the knot by pulling the lock suture with the right hand while maintaining tension on the rail limb with the left hand (Fig. 13.1p). Engage both limbs of the suture with the suture cutter (Fig. 13.1q), advance the cutter below the skin till there is resistance, and then cut the sutures.

StarClose SE™ (Abbott Vascular, Abbott Park, IL): Nitinol Clip

Indications

- The vascular access site should be in the common femoral artery.[1]
- The common femoral artery should be at least 5 mm in diameter.
- 5–6 F arteriotomy can be closed.

Contraindications

- Common femoral artery luminal diameter less than 5 mm in diameter
- Significant peripheral vascular disease
  - Significant luminal encroachment
  - More than moderate fluoroscopically visible calcification

Deployment Steps

- Create a 5–7 mm skin incision at the sheath site to accommodate the insertion of the clip delivery tube into the tissue tract.
- Insert the guidewire and exchange the procedural introducer sheath for the StarClose SE exchange sheath (Fig. 13.2a).
- With heel of the left hand on the patient for support, hold the bottom of the sheath hub and insert the distal tip of the flex-guide into the hub using the right hand (Fig. 13.2b).
- Slowly advance the flex-guide down through the exchange sheath. If there is resistance, the exchange sheath may be kinked.

---

[1] This device has been used successfully for closure of superficial femoral artery arteriotomy.

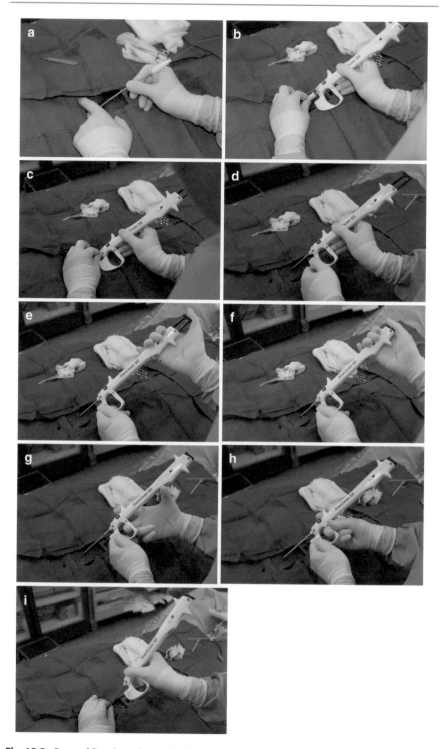

Fig. 13.2 Steps of Starclose closure device deployment

- Connect the clip applier to the sheath hub by pushing the device onto the sheath until it CLICKS into place (Fig. 13.2c).
- With heel of the left hand on the patient for support, grasp the stabilizer to secure the device at the angle of the tissue tract. Pull back the device 2–3 cm (Fig. 13.2d).
- While continuing to stabilize the device with the left hand as described above, assume a "syringe grip" on the proximal end of the device with the right hand by placing the index finger and the middle finger on the proximal posts and the thumb on the plunger (Fig. 13.2e).
- Firmly depress the plunger with the right thumb until it CLICKS into place. The number "2" appears in the number window at this point. This step will deploy the locator wings inside the blood vessel and initiate splitting of the exchange sheath (Fig. 13.2f).
- Check to make sure the number "2" is completely visible in the number window.
- While continuing to stabilize the device with the left hand as described above, switch position of the right hand to a "pistol grip," and gently retract the device with the right hand until slight resistance is felt as the locator wing makes contact with the vessel wall (Fig. 13.2g).
- Fully depress the thumb advancer using the pad of the right thumb until it CLICKS into place. The number "3" appears in the number window at this point (Fig. 13.2h). The clip is resting on the surface of the vessel and is ready to be deployed.
- Raise the body of the device to a 60–75° angle.
- While continuing to stabilize the device with the left hand as described above, switch position of the right hand to a "palm grip." The thumb should rest on the deployment button. Gently push the device down on top of the artery with the right hand to seat the clip delivery tube on top of the access site (Fig. 13.2i) and deploy the device by depressing the deployment button with the right thumb. A final audible click should be heard with device deployment.
- Maintain the downward pressure for 2–3 s. Place the left hand on the puncture site in the palm-down position with the clip delivery tube extending up between the index and middle finger.
- Provide countertraction with the left hand on the patient's body, and remove the device with the right hand.

Angio-Seal™ (St. Jude Medical, St. Paul, MN): Collagen Plug Device

Indications

- The vascular access site should be in the common femoral artery.
- The common femoral artery should be at least 5 mm in diameter.
- 5–6 F arteriotomy can be closed with 6 F Angio-Seal.
- 7–8 F arteriotomy can be closed with 8 F Angio-Seal.

Contraindications

- Common femoral artery luminal diameter less than 5 mm in diameter
- Significant peripheral vascular disease
  - Significant luminal encroachment
  - More than mild fluoroscopically visible calcification

Deployment Steps

- Insert the Angio-Seal guidewire into the procedure sheath.
- Remove the procedure sheath, leaving the guidewire in place to maintain vascular access (Fig. 13.3a).
- Insert the arteriotomy locator into the insertion sheath. If done correctly, the reference indicators (arrows) on the two pieces should match up, and there should subtle click as the two components lock together (Fig. 13.3b). (This step should be performed prior to removal of the procedure sheath.)
- Thread the arteriotomy locator/insertion sheath assembly over the guidewire into the puncture tract. The reference indicators (arrows) on the arteriotomy locator and insertion sheath assembly should be facing up (Fig. 13.3c).
- Advance the assembly until blood begins to flow from the drip hole located near the distal end of the locator (Fig. 13.3d). The blood flow should be brisk, and pulsatile. Once satisfactory backflow of blood is confirmed, pull the assembly back until blood flow stops. Then push the assembly forward again (typically around 1 cm) until brisk blood flow is achieved again. This step ensures that the assembly is not placed too deeply into the artery.
- With the heel of the left hand on the patient for support, hold the insertion sheath with the thumb and forefinger and remove the arteriotomy locator and guidewire (Fig. 13.3e).
- Grasp the TIP of the Angio-Seal device and insert the tip into the delivery sheath. At this point there should be some backflow of blood from around the tip of the device (Fig. 13.3f). (If there is NO flow, then the insertion sheath may have been pulled out of the artery. (Abort the procedure and apply manual pressure for hemostasis.)
- Continue to advance the Angio-Seal device until completely inserted into the insertion sheath and snapped together. There should be an audible click. At this point the reference indicators on the Angio-Seal device and the insertion sheath should match up and should face up (Fig. 13.3g).
- Pull back on the handle of the Angio-Seal device until there is an audible click. The handle of the Angio-Seal device may have to be rocked left and right to ensure that the device is locked in the back position (Fig. 13.3h).
- Pull back on the device handle at the angle of the puncture tract, maintaining a steady uninterrupted motion until there is resistance (Fig. 13.3i). As soon as the delivery suture and a green tamper on the suture becomes visible, advance the tamper while maintaining tension on the suture until resistance against vessel wall is felt and in most cases a black compaction marker is revealed (Fig. 13.3j).

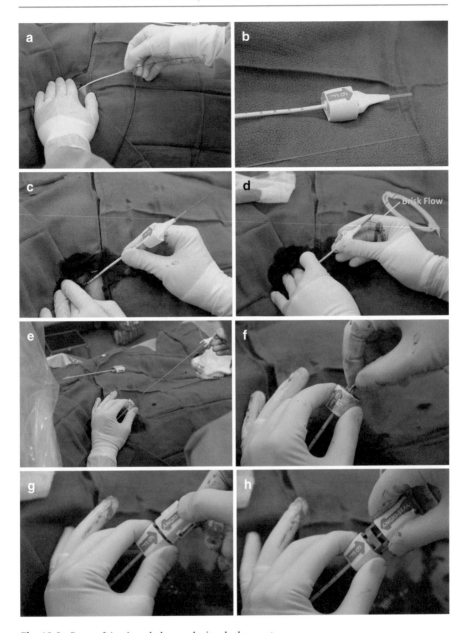

Fig. 13.3 Steps of Angioseal closure device deployment

- Cut the delivery thread below the clear stopper (Fig. 13.3k). Then push down on the skin using a blunt-tip sterile scissor and cut the suture below the skin level (Fig. 13.3l).
- Apply gentle external pressure over the site for 1 min to prevent tract ooze.

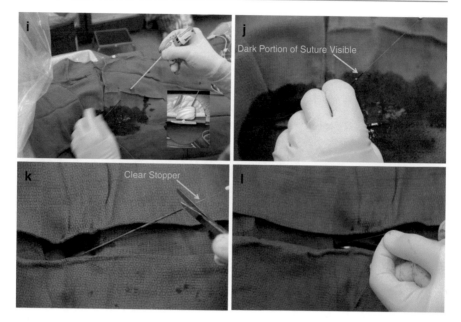

Fig. 13.3 (continued)

MynxGrip™ (AccessClosure, Santa Clara, CA): Polyethylene Glycol Plug Device

Indications

- Common femoral artery punctures.
- Superficial femoral artery punctures.
- Mild peripheral vascular disease.
- 5–7 F arteriotomy can be closed.

Contraindications

- Significant peripheral vascular disease
- Severe calcification proximal to or at the arterial puncture site

Deployment Steps

- Insert MynxGrip into the procedural sheath up to the white shaft marker (Fig. 13.4a).
- Inflate the anchor balloon with about 2 cc of saline with supplied locking syringe until the black marker is fully visible on the inflation indicator and close the device stopcock so that the balloon stays inflated in the vessel (Fig. 13.4b). Leave the syringe on the device stopcock.

- Grasp handle and withdraw catheter until the balloon abuts the distal tip of the procedural sheath. The operator will feel resistance at this point.
- Continue to withdraw the balloon catheter until the balloon abuts the arteriotomy site (Figure Inset). The operator should feel a second point of resistance (Fig. 13.4c). Do NOT continue to pull back. Open the procedural sheath stopcock – there should be no backflow of blood.

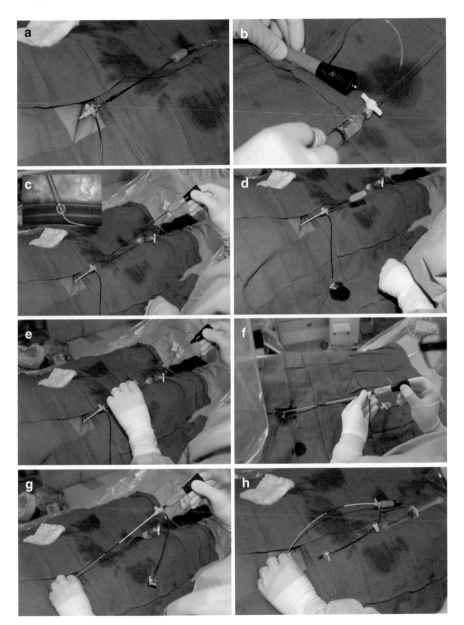

Fig. 13.4 Steps of Mynx closure device deployment

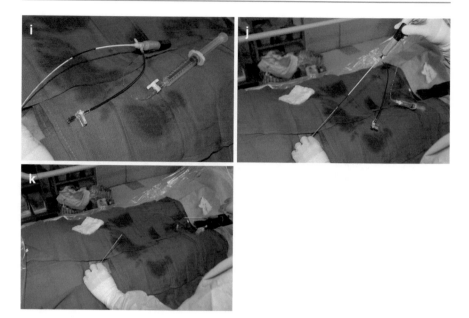

Fig. 13.4 (continued)

- At this point slight relaxation of tension will cause backflow of blood from the procedural sheath stopcock. Reapplication of tension will stop the backflow (Fig. 13.4d). This maneuver confirms that the balloon is in correct position and is abutting the anterior surface of the vessel at the arteriotomy site.
- While lightly holding the device handle to maintain adequate tension on the balloon catheter, detach the shuttle and advance it until resistance is felt (Fig. 13.4e).
- Grasp the procedural sheath and withdraw it from tissue tract. Continue retracting until the shuttle locks on handle (Fig. 13.4f).
- Immediately grasp the advancer tube at the skin and gently advance until the green marker is visible. This step must be performed immediately because the PEG plug must be delivered to the vessel surface before it starts to expand (Fig. 13.4g).
- Lay the device down hold this position for 30 s (Fig. 13.4h). This delay will ensure full expansion of the PEG on the vessel surface.
- Lock the syringe on the device stopcock to max negative, and apply light fingertip compression proximal to the insertion site. Open stopcock to deflate the balloon. To ensure complete balloon deflation, wait until air bubbles and fluid have stopped moving through the inflation tubing (Fig. 13.4i).
- Lightly grasp the advancer tube at the skin with thumb and forefinger and realign with the tissue tract (Fig. 13.4j).
- Slowly withdraw balloon catheter through the advancer tube lumen while holding the advancer tube (Fig. 13.4k).
- Remove advancer tube from the tissue tract. Fingertip compression can be applied for up to 2 min as needed.

Transradial Band™ (Terumo Interventional Systems, Somerset, NJ): Nonocclusive Radial External Hemostasis Device

Indications

- Radial artery punctures.
- 5–7 F arteriotomy can be closed.

Deployment Steps

- Choose appropriate TR Band size (regular or large).
- Pull the access sheath midway back through the arteriotomy site (Fig. 13.5a).
- Wrap TR Band around wrist and secure in place via the Velcro band (Fig. 13.5b).
- For proper positioning the green marker on the translucent band should be placed proximal to the percutaneous access site (Fig. 13.5c).
- Instill 15 cc of air (Fig. 13.5d). Completely remove the sheath then remove air 1 cc at a time until bleeding occurs at which time 1–2 cc of air is reinjected into the balloon. At this point the radial distal to the device should be palpable. The idea is to achieve hemostasis without completing occluding the radial artery.
- Save the syringe for future deflation.
- Approximately 2 h after the sheath is pulled (4 h for PCI), air removal can begin.
- Withdraw 1 cc of air at a time utilizing the provided syringe and observe for any bleeding.

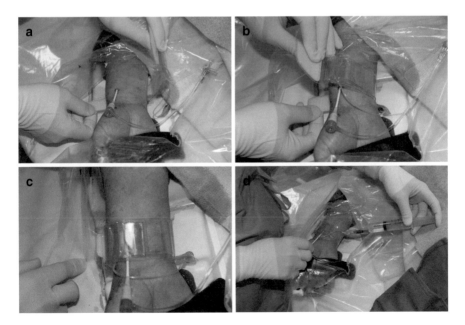

Fig. 13.5 Steps of TR band deployment

- If bleeding occurs reinject air that was removed until hemostasis is achieved, and reattempt deflation in 30 min.
- If no bleeding is observed, the operator should remove all air and deflate the balloon completely and observe for bleeding. If there is no bleeding, the operator can remove the TR Band and place a protective covering (e.g., Tegaderm) over the radial percutaneous site.
- Vital signs and pulse check should be performed every 15 min for the first hour while TR Band is in place, every 30 min during the second hour, and on hourly basis thereafter until post sheath removal. Assess for presence of feeling in the fingers and capillary refill in distal fingers and nail beds until TR Band is removed.

FemoStop™ Mechanical External Compression Device (St. Jude Medical, St. Paul, MN)

Indications

- *Secondary* hemostatic aid for femoral artery access site after delivery of a vascular closure device
- *Secondary* hemostatic aid for femoral artery access site after manual compression
- Hemostatic aid for femoral artery access site oozing or minor bleeding

Contraindications

- Significant peripheral vascular disease.
- Poorly controlled hypertension.
- Uncooperative patient.
- This device should NOT be used as a primary hemostatic device; e.g., this device should not be placed as the only hemostatic measure after pulling a sheath.

Deployment Steps

- Place the band on the bed prior to transitioning patient over on top of it (Fig. 13.6a).
- Place the dome of the FemoStop to cover the arteriotomy site (Fig. 13.6b).
- Make sure FemoStop is positioned in a manner to apply direct vertical pressure down over arteriotomy site (Fig. 13.6c).
- Increase pressure in dome to approximately 20 mmHg above patient's systolic blood pressure and maintain for 3 min (Fig. 13.6d).
- Next reduce pressure to mean arterial pressure over next 5 min, and document distal pulses have not become compromised by this pressure level (Fig. 13.6e).
- Gradually reduce dome pressure over the next 1–1.5 h until device can be safely removed.

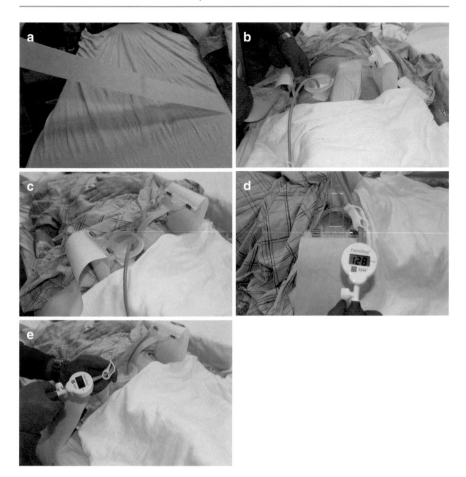

Fig. 13.6 (**a**) Place the band on the bed. (**b**) Place the dome of the Femstop over the arteriotomy site. (**c**) Pull on the side till the device is taut. (**d**) Inflate to 20 mm Hg above patients SBP. (**e**) Reduce the pressure to MAP and ensure distal pulses are felt

- We recommend that this device is not placed overnight. Prolonged use of this device has been associated with arterial leg ischemia as well as formation of deep venous thrombus.

References

1. Caputo RP. Currently approved vascular closure devices. Cardiac Interv Today. 2013; 159(10):660–6.
2. Schwartz BG et al. Review of vascular closure devices. J Invasive Cardiol. 2010;22(12): 599–607.
3. Byrne RA et al. Vascular access and closure in coronary angiography and percutaneous intervention. Nat Rev Cardiol. 2013;10(1):27–40.

Part II

Coronary Intervention

Basics of Intervention

14

Anitha Rajamanickam and Annapoorna Kini

Preprocedural evaluation (focused history, physical examination, stress test and risk grading, evaluating the appropriateness for coronary intervention) and adequate postprocedural care are critical for both procedural and clinical success.

Preprocedural Evaluation Components

History

- Current symptoms, presentation, and angina classification.
- Any symptoms of heart failure.
- History of any cardiac procedures – in patients with known preexisting coronary artery disease, a comprehensive information of all prior catheterizations, percutaneous interventions and cardiac surgeries is vital. Review of prior angiograms to identify location of prior bypass graft origins and type of catheters/devices used is important.
- PVD – information regarding prior peripheral vascular interventions and surgeries is also vital in planning access as is history of claudication.
- CKD – identify patients at risk for contrast-induced nephropathy.
- Smoking, alcohol and substance abuse history, and possibility of withdrawal.
- History of obstructive sleep apnea and lung disorders in regard to the effects of sedation.

A. Rajamanickam, MD (✉) • A. Kini, MD, MRCP, FACC
Department of Interventional Cardiology, Mount Sinai Hospital,
One Gustave Levy Place, Madison Avenue, New York 10029, NY, USA
e-mail: arajamanickam@gmail.com, Anitha.Rajamanickam@mountsinai.org;
Annapoorna.kini@mountsinai.org

© Springer-Verlag London 2014
A. Kini et al. (eds.), *Practical Manual of Interventional Cardiology*,
DOI 10.1007/978-1-4471-6581-1_14

- Ability to take dual antiplatelet therapy and any surgeries/procedures planned within the next year to decide on the type of stent that can be inserted.
- Any history of prior allergic reactions.

Focused physical examination

- Height, weight, body mass index.
- Blood pressure [BP], heart rate [HR], and pulse oximetry.
- Signs of HF [rales, JVD, edema].
- Focused neurological exam.
- Peripheral bilateral lower extremity pulses must be documented.
- Allen and Barbeau's test if radial access is planned.

Prior studies

- Old labs and EKG if available as a baseline for future comparisions.
- Prior PCI, CT surgery reports or CABG reports.
- Prior echocardiogram if available.
- Stress test and risk grading of stress test (see Chap. 5).

Informed consent

Informed consent, risks, benefits, and alternatives of the procedure are explained in layman's terms to the patient. A documentation of the following should be in the patient's chart prior to procedure. "The risks, benefits, and alternatives of cardiac catheterizations/interventions including but not limited to neurovascular trauma, MI, CABG, or death were explained to the patient and/or designated power of attorney. They entirely understand the procedure and have signed the informed consent" (see Table 14.1).

Table 14.1 Major complications of PCI

Complications from NCDR CathPCI Registry	NCDR CathPCI Registry	Mount Sinai Heart
	2010 –July 2012	2010–2012
2010 through July 2012	$n = 787,980$ [1]	$n = 14,584$
Any adverse event	1.53 %	1.0 %
Cardiogenic shock	0.47 %	0.08 %
Pericardial tamponade	0.07 %	0.08 %
CVA/stroke	0.17 %	0.05 %
New requirement for dialysis	0.19 %	0.01 %
Emergent CABG performed during admission	0.17 %	0.02 %
Any vascular complication requiring treatment	0.44 %	0.09 %

Contraindications

There are no absolute contradictions to cardiac catheterization/PCI in acute STEMI/
cardiogenic shock other than patient refusal or inadequate equipment or cardiac
catheterization facility. As most procedures are elective, the patient can be resched-
uled if they have the following:

- Acute flares of other systemic disorders
- Active infection/septic shock
- Acute gastrointestinal bleeding or severe anemia which has not been worked up
- Electrolyte imbalance
- Pregnancy
- Recent cerebrovascular accident (<1 month)
- Rising creatinine but patient not on dialysis
- Acute exacerbation of congestive heart failure
- INR > 3.5 for radial or INR > 2.5 for femoral
- Alcohol intoxication or acute substance abuse

Preprocedural Preparation

- Patient and family teaching (procedure, results, complications).
- Labs:
  - Type and cross match
  - Complete blood cell and platelet counts
  - Prothrombin time [PT], partial thromboplastin time [PTT]
  - Electrolytes, blood urea nitrogen [BUN], creatinine
- 12-lead ECG.
- One or two peripheral IV lines
- Skin-shave and prepare both inguinal areas or the wrist for radial artery.
- *Dietary status*, NPO for at least 4 h:
  - Patients scheduled for morning to noon procedures should be NPO since mid-
    night except for scheduled medications.
  - Patients scheduled for afternoon procedures should have a full breakfast and
    then placed NPO except for scheduled medications.
  - Patients scheduled for evening procedures should have a full breakfast and
    lunch and then placed NPO except for scheduled medications.
- *Allergic reactions*:
  - *Aspirin allergy and aspirin desensitization:* Allergic reactions to aspirin
    include aspirin-exacerbated respiratory disease and angioedema. As dual
    antiplatelet therapy is required in all patients receiving stents for at least 1
    month up to 1 year or longer, aspirin desensitization in aspirin-allergic patients
    should be performed. This can be completed in a day in conjunction with an
    allergist/immunologist in CCU/general cardiology ward or over a few days to
    a week as an outpatient.

Table 14.2 Preprocedural hydration

Start hydration with normal saline [0.9NS] 3 h prior to procedure if outpatient and 12 h prior if inpatient	
LVEF	For all patients but especially if SCr >1.3
>50	1–2 mL/kg/h
31–50	0.5 mL/kg/h
<30	0.3 mL/kg/h for 3 h only for all patients

Table 14.3 Intraprocedural and postprocedural hydration

Continue hydration with normal saline [0.9 NS] during procedure and for 6–8 h post procedure if outpatient and 12 h if inpatient	
LVEF	For all patients but especially if SCr >1.3. If SCr <1.3, IVF can be given for a shorter duration with liberal discharge oral hydration
>50	1–2 mL/kg/h
<50	Measure LVEDP in the catheterization lab. Give a bolus of NS as per LVEDP
	<12: 500 cc
	12–18: 250 cc
	>18: no bolus
31–50	0.5 mL/kg/h
<30	0.3 mL/kg/h

- *Contrast allergy*, all patients reporting true allergy to contrast media should be premedicated. Seafood allergy does not require pretreatment:
  - Prednisone 40 mg orally (or hydrocortisone 100 mg IV/methylprednisolone 40 mg IV) the night prior and on the day of the procedure
  - Antihistamines (Benadryl 25–50 mg orally or IV the night prior and the morning of the procedure
- *Medications on procedure day*:
  - Aspirin 162 mg orally.
  - Continue patient's regular antihypertensive medications, statins, and immunosuppressive medications.
  - Hold oral hypoglycemic medications.
  - Usual dose of basal insulin or a half to one-third dose of NPH insulin can be given on the morning of procedure. Hold short-acting insulin.
- *Hydration* (see Tables 14.2 and 14.3).

Vitals

BP, HR, and pulse oximetry are documented at the start of procedure, every 5 min. continuously during procedure, and every 15 min post procedure for the first 2 h and hourly thereafter.

Medications

- Conscious sedation
  - Versed (midazolam): start with 0.5 mg IV in the elderly and patients with systemic diseases and 1–2 mg in other patients and then as needed to achieve sedation.
  - Morphine sulfate for analgesia: 2–4 mg IV to start and then as needed.
  - Meperidine for patients with morphine allergy: 50–150 mg given 30–90 min before the beginning of anesthesia either subcutaneously or intramuscularly.
  - Acetaminophen: 1 g IV to reduce the need for narcotic analgesia.
  - Metoclopramide: 5 mg IV to prevent opiate-induced nausea.
- Antidotes for conscious sedation:
  - Flumazenil: 0.2 mg over 15 s and repeat doses at 1 min intervals if required to a maximum of 1 mg. In the event of resedation, 0.2 mg at 20 min intervals as needed to a maximum of 3 mg/h.
  - Naloxone: 0.4–2 mg and repeat doses at 2 min intervals if required to a maximum of 10 mg. If no response after 10 mg total, consider other causes of respiratory depression.
- Anticoagulation for diagnostic procedures
  - Heparin: 1,500–2,000 U in patients with prior CABG prior to engagement of grafts or in patients with severe aortic stenosis prior to crossing the valve.
  - Heparin 2,500 U in radial access.
  - If heparin needs to be reversed use:
    - 1 mg of protamine for every 100 U of heparin [maximum dose is 50 mg]
    - 0.5 mg protamine/100 U of heparin if heparin was discontinued 30 min to 1 h prior to procedure
    - 0.25 mg protamine/100 U of heparin if heparin was stopped over 2 h prior to procedure
- Anticoagulation and antithrombotic regimens during PCI (Chap. 5):
  - Bivalirudin: bolus (0.75 mg/kg) and continuous infusion (1.75 mg/kg/h). If creatinine clearance is <30 ml/min, bolus dose remains the same, but infusion dose is reduced to 1 mg/kg/h or 0.25 mg/kg/h if on dialysis. If ACT < 250 3 min after bolus, administer additional 1/2 bolus of bivalirudin or administer additional 1/3 bolus if ACT is 251–299.
  - ReoPro: single bolus only [per nomogram].
  - Integrilin: 1–2 boluses of 180 mcg/kg intravenously 10 min apart in PCIs of very complex lesions, edge dissections, side branch closures, slow flow, no reflows, embolizations, or thrombi.
  - If PCI is planned, load patient with:
    - Clopidogrel – 600 mg if clopidogrel naïve [<5 days on clopidogrel] or 300 mg if on daily maintenance of clopidogrel].
    - Prasugrel – 60 mg if prasugrel naïve or 30 mg if on daily maintenance of prasugrel. Contraindications are active pathological bleeding, prior TIA or stroke, hypersensitivity to prasugrel, and age >75. If switching from clopidogrel to prasugrel, then give 30 mg of prasugrel.

- Ticagrelor – 180 mg if ticagrelor naïve or 90 mg if on daily maintenance of ticagrelor. Contraindications are hypersensitivity to ticagrelor, active pathological bleeding, history of intracranial hemorrhage, and severe hepatic impairment. If switching from Clopidogrel to Ticagrelor give 180 mg of Ticagrelor.
  - Anticoagulation for diagnostic procedures
- IC nitroglycerin for more accurate stenosis severity visualization: 100–200 mcg boluses. If hypotension occurs, administer IV fluid boluses if no volume overload or congestive heart failure is present. Avoid in patients with severe AS. It is contraindicated in right ventricular infraction or after recent use of sidenafil/vardenafil (<24 hrs) or tadalafil (<48 hrs).
  Mix: 25 mg in 250 D5W solution = 100 mcg/ml. Use proper medication bottle/tubing.
- IC verapamil: for SVG graft stenosis/slow flow, 250–500 mcg boluses. Monitor for bradycardia.
  Mix: 1 ml = 2.5 mg, dilute in 10 mL NS syringe = 250 mcg/ml
- IC nitroprusside for slow flow: up to 50–100 mcg or as needed.
  Mix: 12.5 mg in 250 mL D5W solution = 50 mcg/mL. Cover the medication bottle with dark plastic bag to retain medication potency.
- IC phenylephrine: 100–200 mcg boluses. Give 100 mcg IV (1 mL) initially followed by NS flush. Monitor for bradycardia. Higher dosage may cause nausea and may require intravenous metoclopramide or ondansetron.
  Mix: 1 mg in 10 mL NS solution; 100 mcg = 1 mL.

Equipment

- *Vascular access* (please refer to Chap. 2)
- *Temporary pacemaker insertion* (4 F) via 5Fr sheath prior to the procedure in:
  - Complex interventions, use of rotablation or Angiojet mechanical thrombectomy in dominant RCA/LCX
  - The last remaining vessel supplying collaterals to the AV nodal artery
  - BAV
  - Alcohol septal ablation
  - TAVR
- *Guide catheter preparation* (please refer to Chap. 7)
- *Guidewire Shaping* (please refer to Chap. 8)
  - Shaping the wire:
    - C curve for LAD and RCA.
    - L curve for LCX.
    - 1–2 mm sharp angle CTO curves.
    - Another alternative is double curve (primary for the branch, secondary for main vessel).
  - Crossing the lesion with the guidewire:
    - Wiggle the wire.

- Avoid 360° turns.
- Avoid end loop before crossing the lesion.
- Take end loop after crossing the lesion.
- Please refer to Chapter 10: Intracoronary devices for balloon selection and dilatation.
  - Pre-stent deployment: 8–12 atm
  - Stent deployment: 10–12 atm
  - Post-stent deployment: 16–20 atm
- Evaluation of the acute angiographic outcome:
  - Inflow
  - Outflow
  - Dissection
  - Any under-expansion
  - Uncovered area

Postprocedural Considerations

Bed rest

- Coronary angiogram [no AC] with successful VCD deployment: 2 h
- Coronary angiogram [no AC] with manual hold hemostasis: [sheath size-2] hours
- PCI with successful VCD deployment: 2 h post discontinuation of anticoagulation
- PCI with manual hold hemostasis: [sheath size-1] hours after sheath removal

Fluids   Continue as per Table 14.2.

Labs

- CBC, BMP, and troponin I at 3–6 h in all patients and subsequently if there are any lab abnormalities
- CBC, BMP, and troponin I at 12–18 h if monitored overnight and subsequently if there are any laboratory abnormalities

Imaging

- *EKG:* 3–6 h after procedure and subsequently as per symptoms
- *Echo:* after NSTEMI/STEMI to evaluate LV function if a ventriculogram is not performed

Disposition after the procedure

- Diagnostic procedure – same day discharge:
  - 2 h discharge if closure device was used successfully
  - 4 h discharge if manual compression hemostasis was achieved (5–6 Fr sheaths)

- Simple PCI – same day discharge:
  - 4–6 h if closure device was used successfully
  - 6–8 h if manual compression hemostasis was achieved
- Inpatient admission – any patient who needs inpatient monitoring:
  - Presentation as STEMI or non-STEMI or hemodynamic instability (cardiogenic shock, CHF, significant brady- or tachyarrhythmia)
  - Major vascular complications:
  - Age > 85 years
  - Significant comorbid conditions:
    - Ventricular arrhythmia or rapid atrial arrhythmia
    - Decompensated systolic heart failure or LVEF <30 %
    - Chronic renal insufficiency (SCr ≥ 1.8 mg/dl)
    - Prior organ transplant or immunosuppressive state
  - Complex or high-risk coronary intervention such as:
    - Unprotected LM or LM equivalent
    - Vein or arterial graft intervention
    - Bifurcation lesion requiring both branch interventions
    - Use of atherectomy devices
    - Use of thrombectomy devices
    - CTO requiring bilateral injection
    - Prolonged procedure with fluoro time >60 min
  - Procedural complications such as:
    - No flow/slow flow
    - Side branch closure
    - Perforation
    - Residual dissection [type C or more]
    - Thromboembolism
    - Postprocedural chest pain or EKG changes
    - Hemodynamic instability requiring treatment
    - Elevated cardiac enzymes: CK-MB >3 × baseline
  - Inability to ambulate due to:
    - Poor coordination
    - Vasomotor instability
    - Dizziness or suspected neurological issues/events
  - High-risk patients requiring therapeutic long-term anticoagulation
  - No social support or inability to get access to medical care in case of an emergency

Post-PTCA pharmacology

- Hold metformin for 48 h post procedure.
- Dual antiplatelet therapy for at least 4 weeks after stenting with a bare metal stent and 12 months with a drug-eluting stent.

- Start high dose statin therapy.
- Evaluate the need for cardiac rehabilitation.
- Smoking cessation counseling in indicated patients.
- Dietary counseling and risk factor/life style modification.
- Anti-anginal therapy and maximal medical management as indicated by current guidelines.

Reference

1. Dehmer GJ, Weaver D, Roe MT, Milford-Beland S, Fitzgerald S, Hermann A, Messenger J, Moussa I, Garratt K, Rumsfeld J, Brindis RG. A contemporary view of diagnostic cardiac catheterization and percutaneous coronary intervention in the United States: a report from the CathPCI Registry of the National Cardiovascular Data Registry, 2010 through June 2011. J Am Coll Cardiol. 2012;60(20):2017–31. doi:10.1016/j.jacc.2012.08.966. Epub 2012 Oct 17. PubMed PMID: 23083784.

Difficult Stent Delivery

15

Anitha Rajamanickam and Annapoorna Kini

Stent delivery remains challenging in around 5 % of PCIs, despite gigantic technical advances in the field of interventional cardiology. Unsuccessful stent placement is associated with inferior short term and long term outcomes. Failure of stent deployment may lead to stent embolization during withdrawal maneuvers.

Characteristics Associated with Stent Delivery Failure

- Vessel tortuosity – iliac, femoral, and coronary
- Lesion severity
- Lesion length
- Coronary calcifications (before and at the lesion)
- Stent length
- Poor guiding catheter support

Steps to Prevent Difficulties in Stent Delivery

- Long sheath
- Appropriate guide selection

A. Rajamanickam, MD (✉) • A. Kini, MD, MRCP, FACC
Department of Interventional Cardiology, Mount Sinai Hospital,
One Gustave Levy Place, Madison Avenue, New York 10029, NY, USA
e-mail: arajamanickam@gmail.com, Anitha.Rajamanickam@mountsinai.org;
Annapoorna.kini@mountsinai.org

© Springer-Verlag London 2014
A. Kini et al. (eds.), *Practical Manual of Interventional Cardiology*,
DOI 10.1007/978-1-4471-6581-1_15

- Lesion preparation/plaque modification
  - Low-profile balloon
  - High-pressure NC balloon
  - Cutting balloon or atherectomy devices

Steps to Help with Difficult Stent Delivery

- Deep seating the guide
- Deep inspiration
- Buddy wire or changing the wire
- Guideliner
- Change stent length
- Buddy-in-jail technique
- PTCA alone

Steps to Prevent Difficulties in Stent Delivery

Long sheath Anticipate the need for a long sheath. Rotations and manipulations at the proximal end do not transmit to the distal end of devices and guides in excessively tortuous iliac and femoral arteries. A long sheath will improve guide support. Initially place the sheath tip in the descending aorta and advance further if extra backup is required.

Appropriate guide selection Coaxial engagement is the key and it is imperative to choose the correct guide to provide passive support. Active support is provided by deep seating the guide (see Chap. 7 Guiding Catheter Selection).

Adequate lesion preparation This is the most important step. Adequate predilation with high-pressure balloons or cutting balloons must be performed prior to stent insertion. If you have trouble passing even a small [1.2/8 mm] compliant balloon or a microcatheter, then consider rotational or orbital atherectomy.

Steps to Help with Difficult Stent Delivery

Deep seating guide Deep seating of the guide into the artery improves backup support and pushability of devices regardless of the anatomy of the coronary vessel and the morphology of the lesions. Patients, in whom dissections of the proximal vessel might be likely, such as those with diffuse disease or small proximal vessels, are not ideal candidates for such an approach. Deep seating may later result in ostial stenosis due to endothelial trauma. It is important that the guide is maneuvered into the coronaries over the shaft of a PTCA balloon or stent delivery catheter to minimize this risk.

Deep inspiration The easiest maneuver to try is deep inspiration. During inspiration, the coronary arteries move caudally and the RCA and LAD also tend to move posteriorly. Deep inspiration can reduce vascular tortuosity, particularly within the proximal segments; displaces the diaphragm and heart into a more vertical position; and straightens the coronary tree, enabling an easier device delivery.

Buddy wire A second wire, *buddy wire technique*, may help to straighten the vessel. A variant of the buddy wire technique is the *gliding wire technique*, where a second hydrophilic wire is inserted in order to allow the stent to glide over the hydrophilic coating of the second wire. Another variant is the *anchor wire technique*, where a second wire is inserted in a nontarget vessel of the left system or a branch of the vessel for the right coronary system.

Changing wire Changing wires can prove to be a simple and less expensive strategy for difficult stent delivery. A long stent loaded on a floppy wire may not have enough support for its passage, in which case changing to a firmer wire might be useful. However, in certain cases stents loaded on extra support wire may push against the wall of a heavily calcified and angulated lesion, making the stent passage difficult. Changing to a less firm wire might be helpful in this situation. A microcathter is useful here for changing wires across a difficult-to-cross lesion (see Chap. 8).

- Runthrough™, BMW™, and Luge Prowater™ are examples of firm, non-hydrophilic wires.
- Fielder™, Whisper™, and Choice PT™ are examples of floppy, hydrophilic wires.
- Mailman™ and Grandslam™ are examples of extra support wires.
- Wiggle wire™ is a specialty wire designed to exert a force in a different plane to allow for successful stent/device delivery through a previously deployed stent.

Guideliner™ Mother and child catheter extension (catheter inside a catheter). The Guideliner™ is a 25 cm guide extension connected to a pushrod with a 15 cm "half-pipe" collar (170°) that reduces the potential for wire wrap. It has a tapered closing that directs stent struts away from collar lip. This device allows deep extension into vessel and facilitates backup support and stent delivery, significantly extending the scope of coronary intervention possible within a 6F mother guide catheter (Fig. 15.1). It should be considered either to increase backup support or enable stent delivery when problems are encountered using conventional techniques or upfront in the setting of very complex disease. Sometimes, the Guideliner is advanced deep into the coronary artery with the help of anchor balloon to facilitate stent delivery, especially in delivery of long stents. It is critical that the guideliner is only advanced over a balloon into the coronary artery.

Change stent length A less attractive and expensive option is changing to one or two shorter stents or a different stent type.

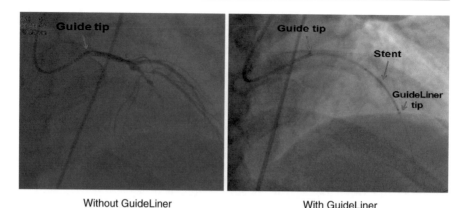

Without GuideLiner   With GuideLiner

Fig. 15.1 Guideliner: deep seating for device placement

Buddy-in-jail technique The buddy-in-jail technique is rarely used. It is useful when standard techniques fail to deliver the stent to a distal stenosis and there is additional proximal stenosis that the interventionalist intends to stent. A second non-hydrophilic coated buddy wire of at least medium support is wired to the distal vessel. The proximal vessel is then stented and the buddy wire is jailed. The jailed in buddy wire provides the support to deliver the distal stent through the proximally placed stent by the following mechanisms:

• The guiding catheter will be anchored more securely within the ostium of the vessel.
• The jailed buddy wire may straighten the proximal portion of the vessel.
• The jailed wire may increase the rigidity of the distal wire segment.

A non-coated buddy wire should be used and the radiopaque portion of the wire should not be jailed. The proximal stent should be deployed using only modest pressure (12 atm or less) to minimize the risk of wire entrapment or fracture. Before deployment of the distal stent, the jailed buddy wire should be removed to avoid "double jailing." The proximal stent must be postdilated at the end.

Settling for PTCA without stent When acceptable, provisional PTCA with results confirmed by intravascular ultrasound or fractional flow reserve may be the best solution for difficult stent delivery.

Bifurcation Lesions

16

Sadik Raja Panwar, Anitha Rajamanickam,
and Annapoorna Kini

Treatment of coronary bifurcation lesions represents an area of ongoing challenge in interventional cardiology. Based on contemporary trials, provisional stenting has better clinical outcomes.

Definition

Bifurcation lesion is defined as a lesion of >50 % involving a bifurcation with a side branch that is ≥1.5 mm in size.

Anatomic Challenges

- Plaque burden of the main vessel and side branch
- Calcification
- Bifurcation angle

Medina bifurcation classification is most commonly used. It is numbered as (x,x,x). Each x is either 0 (<50 % stenosis) or 1 (≥50 % stenosis) and denotes in order the proximal main vessel (PMV), distal main vessel (DMV) and side branch vessel (SBV) [1].

S.R. Panwar, MD • A. Rajamanickam, MD • A. Kini, MD, MRCP, FACC (✉)
Department of Interventional Cardiology, Mount Sinai Hospital,
One Gustave Levy Place, Madison Avenue, New York, NY 10029, USA
e-mail: drsrpanwar@gmail.com; Annapoorna.kini@mountsinai.org,
arajamanickam@gmail.com, Anitha.Rajamanickam@mountsinai.org

© Springer-Verlag London 2014
A. Kini et al. (eds.), *Practical Manual of Interventional Cardiology*,
DOI 10.1007/978-1-4471-6581-1_16

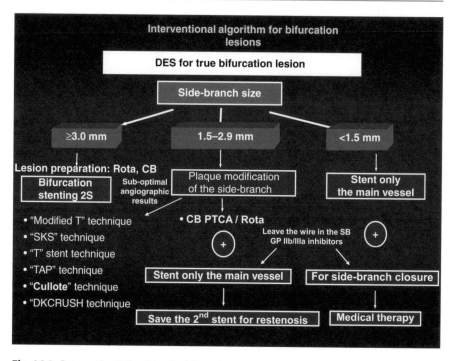

Fig. 16.1 Interventional algorithm for bifurcation coronary lesions

Approach to Bifurcation Intervention

Access

- Femoral or radial:
  6 Fr for provisional stenting approach.
  7 Fr Guide is required for most of the dedicated 2 stent strategies.
  A 45 cm long sheath is preferred as it provides extra support.

Guiding Catheter Selection

LCA bifurcation lesions	Provisional: 6 Fr VL/EBU guide
	Dedicated 2 stent: 7 Fr VL/EBU guide
RCA bifurcation lesions	Provisional: 6 Fr AR 2 or AL 0.75
	Dedicated 2 stent: 7 Fr AR 2 or AL 0.75

Optimal Views

- *Distal left main:* LAO Caudal (30–60°, 25–30°)
- *LAD/diagonal bifurcation:* RAO cranial (10°,40°)
- *Diagonol ostium visualization:* LAO cranial (40–45°, 25–30°)
- *For early diagonals:* LAO caudal (45–55°, 25–30°)
- *LCX/marginal:* AP caudal (0, 25°–40°), and LAO caudal (45–55°, 25–30°)
- *Distal RCA/ RPDA:* AP/LAO Cranial (0–55°, 30°)

Wiring

- Hydrophilic wires (eg. Fielder™) is preferred for side branch vessel [SBV]
- Wiring, and a workhorse wire (eg. Runthrough™) is preferred for main branch [MBV] wiring.
- The more complex lesion should be wired first.
- When wiring the second vessel, avoid excessive torquing and 360° turns. Use small side to side movements in order to prevent intertwining.

Lesion Preparation

- Adequate lesion preparation is essential. Use of cutting balloons and atherectomy devices may be essential is severely calcified lesions.

Provisional Stenting Approach

- First perform MBV predilation.
- Assess for plaque shift into SBV. If there is plaque shift and TIMI 3 flow is compromized perform PTCA [1:1 sizing] or CB PTCA [1/4 size smaller than reference vessel] of the SBV.
- Reassess side branch. If there is no plaque shift and TIMI 3 flow is preserved proceed with provisional stenting of the MBV [nominal pressure] with a wire in the SBV.
- Remove the jailed SBV wire. If high-pressure balloon postdilation of the MBV stent is required, rewire the SBV and perform postdialtion.
- Reassess side branch again. If patient is chest-pain-free and there is TIMI III flow in SBV, take final angiogram; otherwise perform kissing balloon technique (KBI) or bailout stenting using the TAP technique [see below].
- KBI: Initially perform PTCA of jailed side branch using complaint balloon [1:1 sizing] to open the stent struts. If difficulty is encountered, use a smaller complaint balloon to open the stent struts. Perform final KBI with NC balloon in the MBV [1:1 sizing] and compliant balloon in SBV [1:1 sizing].

Two-Stent Approach

- MBV and SBV predilation. PTCA of more severe stenosis is preferably performed first. Stenting strategy will depend on the anatomical characteristics as described below:
  - *SKS:* Preferred for Medina [1,1,1]. The two stents overlap of 3 mm or more in the MBV. This requires the MBV diameter to be atleast 2/3rd the size of sum of the DBV and SBV diameters (Fig. 16.2).
  - *V-stenting:* Preferred for Medina [0,1,1]. The two stents overlap of 2 mm or less in the MBV (Fig. 16.3).
  - *Routine T-stenting* (Fig. 16.4)/*modified T-stenting* (Fig. 16.5): Usually preferred in Medina(1,1,1) and with a SBV which has origin with angle >70° to around 90°, preferably closer to 90°.

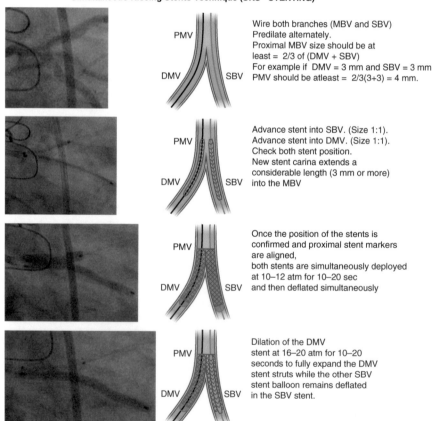

Fig. 16.2 SKS: simultaneous kissing stent technique

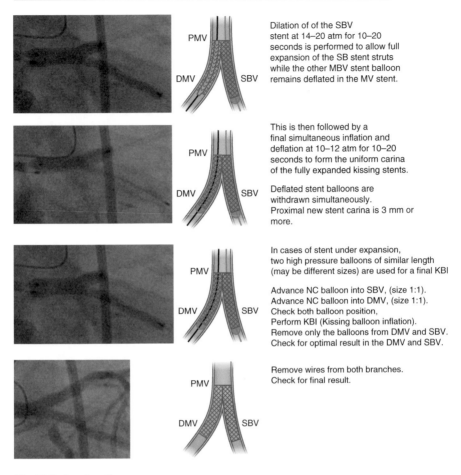

Dilation of of the SBV stent at 14–20 atm for 10–20 seconds is performed to allow full expansion of the SB stent struts while the other MBV stent balloon remains deflated in the MV stent.

This is then followed by a final simultaneous inflation and deflation at 10–12 atm for 10–20 seconds to form the uniform carina of the fully expanded kissing stents.

Deflated stent balloons are withdrawn simultaneously. Proximal new stent carina is 3 mm or more.

In cases of stent under expansion, two high pressure balloons of similar length (may be different sizes) are used for a final KBI

Advance NC balloon into SBV, (size 1:1). Advance NC balloon into DMV, (size 1:1). Check both balloon position, Perform KBI (Kissing balloon inflation). Remove only the balloons from DMV and SBV. Check for optimal result in the DMV and SBV.

Remove wires from both branches. Check for final result.

Fig. 16.2 (continued)

- *Mini-crush:* Usually preferred in Medina(1,1,1) and with a SBV which has origin with angle <70° (Fig. 16.6).
- *Culotte:* Preferred for large MBV and SBV in Medina (1,1,1) and with a SBV which has origin with angle <70° (Fig. 16.7).
- *DK crush:* in Medina(1,1,1) and can be performed with 6 Fr guide (Fig. 16.8).
- *T and protrusion [TAP]* (Fig. 16.9)/*reverse crush* (Fig. 16.10)*:* Bailout stenting strategy for provisional approach.

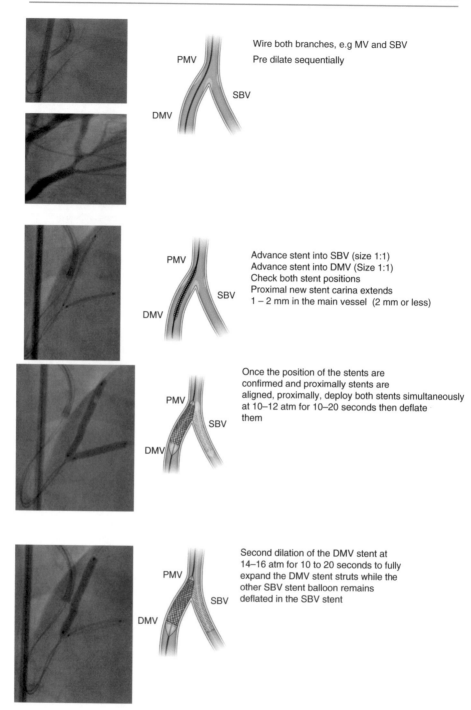

Wire both branches, e.g MV and SBV
Pre dilate sequentially

Advance stent into SBV (size 1:1)
Advance stent into DMV (Size 1:1)
Check both stent positions
Proximal new stent carina extends
1 – 2 mm in the main vessel (2 mm or less)

Once the position of the stents are
confirmed and proximally stents are
aligned, proximally, deploy both stents simultaneously
at 10–12 atm for 10–20 seconds then deflate
them

Second dilation of the DMV stent at
14–16 atm for 10 to 20 seconds to fully
expand the DMV stent struts while the
other SBV stent balloon remains
deflated in the SBV stent

Fig. 16.3 V-stenting steps similar to SKS with proximal new stent carina that extends 2 mm or less

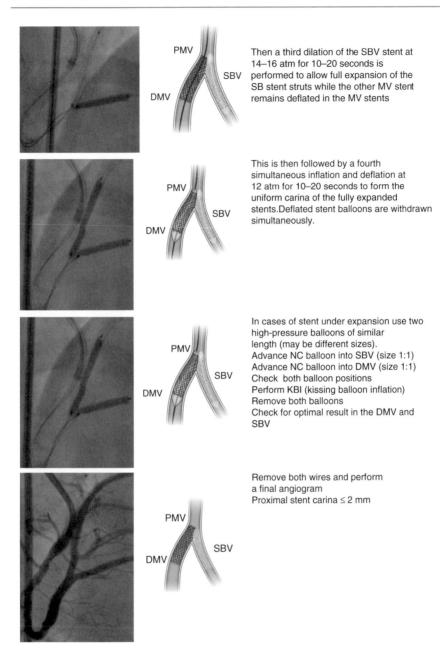

Then a third dilation of the SBV stent at 14–16 atm for 10–20 seconds is performed to allow full expansion of the SB stent struts while the other MV stent remains deflated in the MV stents

This is then followed by a fourth simultaneous inflation and deflation at 12 atm for 10–20 seconds to form the uniform carina of the fully expanded stents.Deflated stent balloons are withdrawn simultaneously.

In cases of stent under expansion use two high-pressure balloons of similar length (may be different sizes).
Advance NC balloon into SBV (size 1:1)
Advance NC balloon into DMV (size 1:1)
Check both balloon positions
Perform KBI (kissing balloon inflation)
Remove both balloons
Check for optimal result in the DMV and SBV

Remove both wires and perform a final angiogram
Proximal stent carina ≤ 2 mm

Fig. 16.3 (continued)

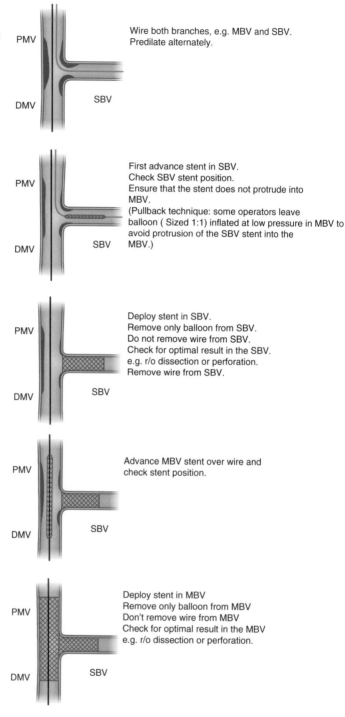

Fig. 16.4 Classic T-stenting or routine T technique

PMV

DMV   SBV

Wire both branches, e.g. MBV and SBV.
Predilate alternately.

First advance stent in SBV.
Check SBV stent position.
Ensure that the stent does not protrude into MBV.
(Pullback technique: some operators leave balloon (Sized 1:1) inflated at low pressure in MBV to avoid protrusion of the SBV stent into the MBV.)

Deploy stent in SBV.
Remove only balloon from SBV.
Do not remove wire from SBV.
Check for optimal result in the SBV.
e.g. r/o dissection or perforation.
Remove wire from SBV.

Advance MBV stent over wire and check stent position.

Deploy stent in MBV
Remove only balloon from MBV
Don't remove wire from MBV
Check for optimal result in the MBV
e.g. r/o dissection or perforation.

Fig. 16.4   (continued)

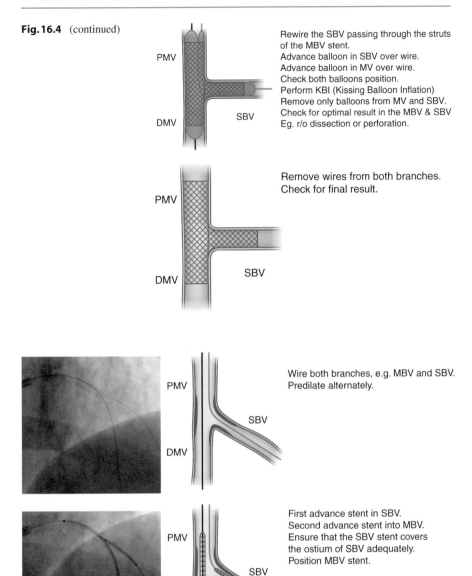

Rewire the SBV passing through the struts
of the MBV stent.
Advance balloon in SBV over wire.
Advance balloon in MV over wire.
Check both balloons position.
Perform KBI (Kissing Balloon Inflation)
Remove only balloons from MV and SBV.
Check for optimal result in the MBV & SBV
Eg. r/o dissection or perforation.

Remove wires from both branches.
Check for final result.

Wire both branches, e.g. MBV and SBV.
Predilate alternately.

First advance stent in SBV.
Second advance stent into MBV.
Ensure that the SBV stent covers
the ostium of SBV adequately.
Position MBV stent.

Fig. 16.5   Modified T-stenting technique

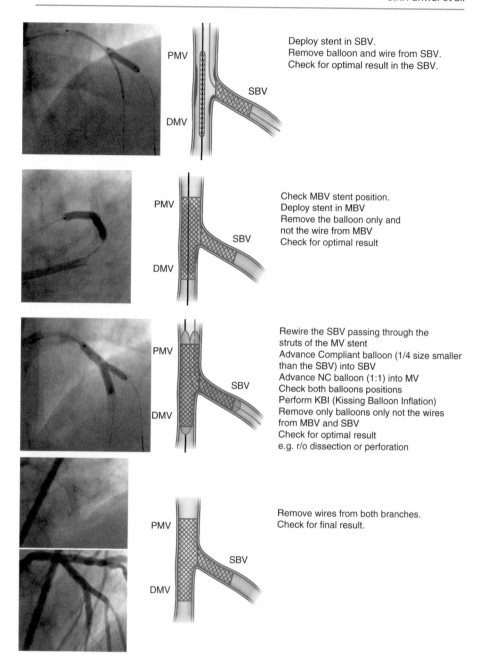

Deploy stent in SBV.
Remove balloon and wire from SBV.
Check for optimal result in the SBV.

Check MBV stent position.
Deploy stent in MBV
Remove the balloon only and
not the wire from MBV
Check for optimal result

Rewire the SBV passing through the
struts of the MV stent
Advance Compliant balloon (1/4 size smaller
than the SBV) into SBV
Advance NC balloon (1:1) into MV
Check both balloons positions
Perform KBI (Kissing Balloon Inflation)
Remove only balloons only not the wires
from MBV and SBV
Check for optimal result
e.g. r/o dissection or perforation

Remove wires from both branches.
Check for final result.

Fig. 16.5 (continued)

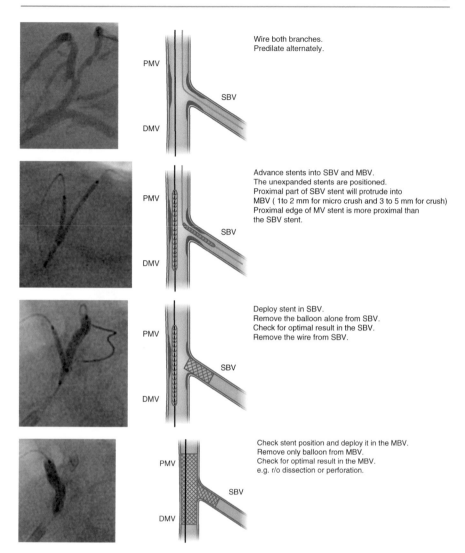

PMV

SBV

DMV

Wire both branches.
Predilate alternately.

PMV

SBV

DMV

Advance stents into SBV and MBV.
The unexpanded stents are positioned.
Proximal part of SBV stent will protrude into
MBV (1to 2 mm for micro crush and 3 to 5 mm for crush)
Proximal edge of MV stent is more proximal than
the SBV stent.

PMV

SBV

DMV

Deploy stent in SBV.
Remove the balloon alone from SBV.
Check for optimal result in the SBV.
Remove the wire from SBV.

PMV

SBV

DMV

Check stent position and deploy it in the MBV.
Remove only balloon from MBV.
Check for optimal result in the MBV.
e.g. r/o dissection or perforation.

Fig. 16.6 Mini-crush technique

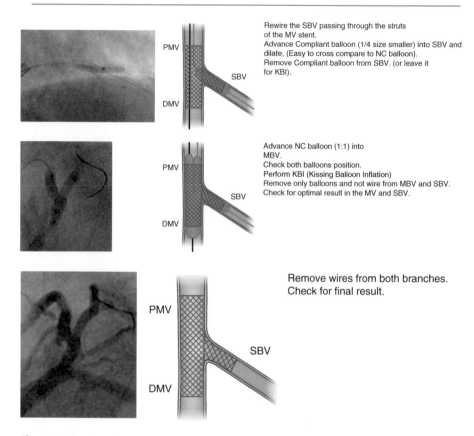

Rewire the SBV passing through the struts of the MV stent.
Advance Compliant balloon (1/4 size smaller) into SBV and dilate, (Easy to cross compare to NC balloon).
Remove Compliant balloon from SBV. (or leave it for KBI).

Advance NC balloon (1:1) into MBV.
Check both balloons position.
Perform KBI (Kissing Balloon Inflation)
Remove only balloons and not wire from MBV and SBV.
Check for optimal result in the MV and SBV.

Remove wires from both branches.
Check for final result.

Fig. 16.6 (continued)

Fig. 16.7 The culotte
stenting technique

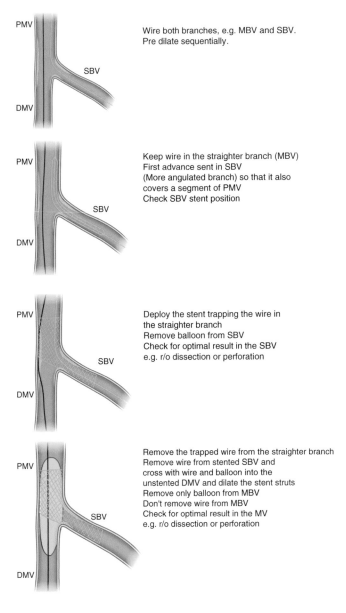

Wire both branches, e.g. MBV and SBV.
Pre dilate sequentially.

Keep wire in the straighter branch (MBV)
First advance sent in SBV
(More angulated branch) so that it also
covers a segment of PMV
Check SBV stent position

Deploy the stent trapping the wire in
the straighter branch
Remove balloon from SBV
Check for optimal result in the SBV
e.g. r/o dissection or perforation

Remove the trapped wire from the straighter branch
Remove wire from stented SBV and
cross with wire and balloon into the
unstented DMV and dilate the stent struts
Remove only balloon from MBV
Don't remove wire from MBV
Check for optimal result in the MV
e.g. r/o dissection or perforation

Fig. 16.7 (continued)

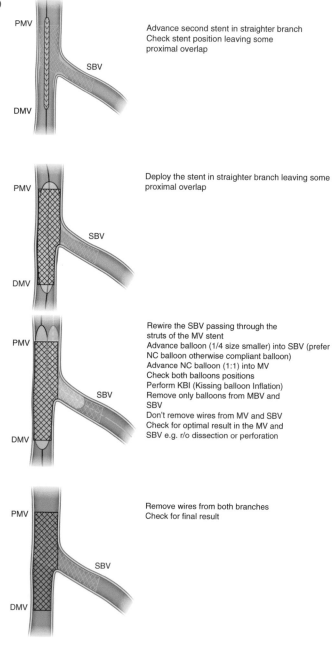

Advance second stent in straighter branch
Check stent position leaving some
proximal overlap

Deploy the stent in straighter branch leaving some
proximal overlap

Rewire the SBV passing through the
struts of the MV stent
Advance balloon (1/4 size smaller) into SBV (prefer
NC balloon otherwise compliant balloon)
Advance NC balloon (1:1) into MV
Check both balloons positions
Perform KBI (Kissing balloon Inflation)
Remove only balloons from MBV and
SBV
Don't remove wires from MV and SBV
Check for optimal result in the MV and
SBV e.g. r/o dissection or perforation

Remove wires from both branches
Check for final result

Fig. 16.8 Double-kissing crush technique (DK crush stenting)

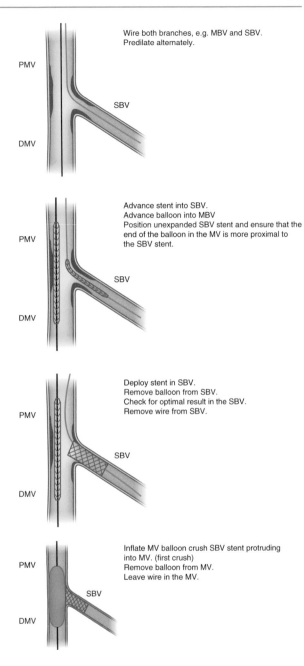

Wire both branches, e.g. MBV and SBV.
Predilate alternately.

PMV

SBV

DMV

Advance stent into SBV.
Advance balloon into MBV
Position unexpanded SBV stent and ensure that the
end of the balloon in the MV is more proximal to
the SBV stent.

PMV

SBV

DMV

Deploy stent in SBV.
Remove balloon from SBV.
Check for optimal result in the SBV.
Remove wire from SBV.

PMV

SBV

DMV

Inflate MV balloon crush SBV stent protruding
into MV. (first crush)
Remove balloon from MV.
Leave wire in the MV.

PMV

SBV

DMV

Fig. 16.8 (continued)

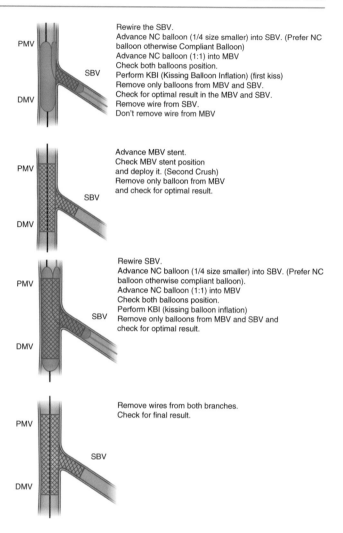

Rewire the SBV.
Advance NC balloon (1/4 size smaller) into SBV. (Prefer NC balloon otherwise Compliant Balloon)
Advance NC balloon (1:1) into MBV
Check both balloons position.
Perform KBI (Kissing Balloon Inflation) (first kiss)
Remove only balloons from MBV and SBV.
Check for optimal result in the MBV and SBV.
Remove wire from SBV.
Don't remove wire from MBV

Advance MBV stent.
Check MBV stent position
and deploy it. (Second Crush)
Remove only balloon from MBV
and check for optimal result.

Rewire SBV.
Advance NC balloon (1/4 size smaller) into SBV. (Prefer NC balloon otherwise compliant balloon).
Advance NC balloon (1:1) into MBV
Check both balloons position.
Perform KBI (kissing balloon inflation)
Remove only balloons from MBV and SBV and check for optimal result.

Remove wires from both branches.
Check for final result.

Fig. 16.9 T-stenting and
small protrusion (TAP)

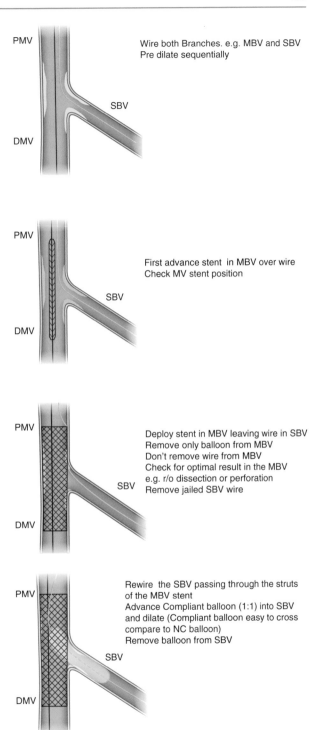

Wire both Branches. e.g. MBV and SBV
Pre dilate sequentially

First advance stent in MBV over wire
Check MV stent position

Deploy stent in MBV leaving wire in SBV
Remove only balloon from MBV
Don't remove wire from MBV
Check for optimal result in the MBV
e.g. r/o dissection or perforation
Remove jailed SBV wire

Rewire the SBV passing through the struts
of the MBV stent
Advance Compliant balloon (1:1) into SBV
and dilate (Compliant balloon easy to cross
compare to NC balloon)
Remove balloon from SBV

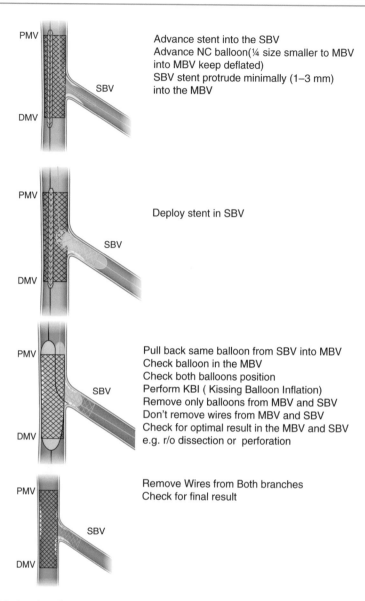

Advance stent into the SBV
Advance NC balloon(¼ size smaller to MBV
into MBV keep deflated)
SBV stent protrude minimally (1–3 mm)
into the MBV

Deploy stent in SBV

Pull back same balloon from SBV into MBV
Check balloon in the MBV
Check both balloons position
Perform KBI (Kissing Balloon Inflation)
Remove only balloons from MBV and SBV
Don't remove wires from MBV and SBV
Check for optimal result in the MBV and SBV
e.g. r/o dissection or perforation

Remove Wires from Both branches
Check for final result

Fig. 16.9 (continued)

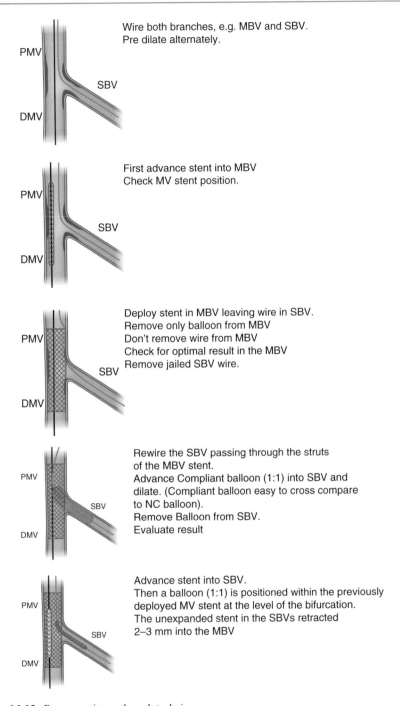

Wire both branches, e.g. MBV and SBV.
Pre dilate alternately.

First advance stent into MBV
Check MV stent position.

Deploy stent in MBV leaving wire in SBV.
Remove only balloon from MBV
Don't remove wire from MBV
Check for optimal result in the MBV
Remove jailed SBV wire.

Rewire the SBV passing through the struts
of the MBV stent.
Advance Compliant balloon (1:1) into SBV and
dilate. (Compliant balloon easy to cross compare
to NC balloon).
Remove Balloon from SBV.
Evaluate result

Advance stent into SBV.
Then a balloon (1:1) is positioned within the previously
deployed MV stent at the level of the bifurcation.
The unexpanded stent in the SBVs retracted
2–3 mm into the MBV

Fig. 16.10 Reverse or internal crush technique

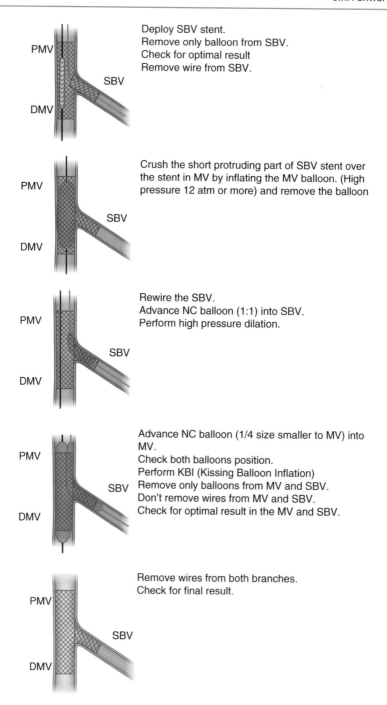

Deploy SBV stent.
Remove only balloon from SBV.
Check for optimal result
Remove wire from SBV.

Crush the short protruding part of SBV stent over the stent in MV by inflating the MV balloon. (High pressure 12 atm or more) and remove the balloon

Rewire the SBV.
Advance NC balloon (1:1) into SBV.
Perform high pressure dilation.

Advance NC balloon (1/4 size smaller to MV) into MV.
Check both balloons position.
Perform KBI (Kissing Balloon Inflation)
Remove only balloons from MV and SBV.
Don't remove wires from MV and SBV.
Check for optimal result in the MV and SBV.

Remove wires from both branches.
Check for final result.

Fig. 16.10 (continued)

References

1. Sharma SK, Choudhury A, Lee J, et al. Simultaneous kissing stents (SKS) technique for treating bifurcation lesions in medium-to-large size coronary arteries. Am J Cardiol. 2004;94:913–7.
2. Pan M, de Lezo JS, Medina A, et al. Rapamycin-eluting stents for the treatment of bifurcated coronary lesions: a randomized comparison of a simple versus complex strategy. Am Heart J. 2004;148:857–64.
3. Colombo A, Stankovic G, Orlic D, et al. Modified T-stenting technique with crushing for bifurcation lesions: immediate results and 30-day outcome. Catheter Cardiovasc Interv. 2003;60:145–51.

Ostial Lesion Interventions

17

Mayur Lakhani, Anitha Rajamanickam,
and Annapoorna Kini

Ostial lesions pose distinctive technical challenges. This chapter provides an overview of equipment and interventional techniques used for ostial lesions.

Definition

- Ostial lesions are defined as lesions within 3 mm of the origin of the vessel. It could be at the aorto-ostial or branch-ostial junction.

Anatomic Challenges

- Inability to engage the guide and maintain position
- High degree of elastic recoil
- High restenosis rate
- Different takeoff angles from aorta
- Difficulty in precise placement using conventional fluoroscopic images is critical. In aorto ostial lesion protrusion into the aorta will cause difficulty during recannalisation. In non aorto ostial lesions "pinching" of the second vessel may occur if placement is not performed.

M. Lakhani, MD (✉) • A. Rajamanickam, MD • A. Kini, MD, MRCP, FACC
Department of Interventional Cardiology, Mount Sinai Hospital,
One Gustave Levy Place, Madison Avenue, New York 10029, NY, USA
e-mail: drmayurlakhani@gmail.com; arajamanickam@gmail.com,
Anitha.rajamanickam@mountsinai.org; Annapoorna.kini@mountsinai.org

© Springer-Verlag London 2014
A. Kini et al. (eds.), *Practical Manual of Interventional Cardiology*,
DOI 10.1007/978-1-4471-6581-1_17

Equipment

- *Sheath:* 6 Fr
- *Guide selection/position:*Choose a less aggressive guide that will provide coaxial alignment without the tendency of deep engagement; this will also facilitate disengagement of the guide during stent placement.
  - Guide catheter with side holes may be preferred in cases of subtotal aorto-ostial lesion.
  - Guide selection will depend on the vessel takeoff and various other factors.
  - For RCA, IM or FR 4 guide with side holes should be used.
  - For LM, FL guides (due to its short tip) with side holes should be used.
  - For RCA bypass grafts, multipurpose or AR2 with side holes should be used.
  - For OM or diagonal grafts, AR 2 or AL1 with side holes should be used.
  - Position: guide should not be fully engaged or deep seated.
  - For severe ostial disease, pre-load the wire in the guide before vessel intubation. This will facilitate rapid wiring and catheter disengagement after wiring.
  - A buddy wire may also be used to provide additional stability or as a marker in the ascending aorta or side branch to assist in positioning the stent.
  - Once the device (balloon, stent, etc.) is positioned, the guide is gently withdrawn into the aorta. Prior to complete removal of the device from the artery, use the device to "rail in" the guide tip (prevents damage to the deployed stent).
- *Wires:* A standard workhorse 0.014″ wire is appropriate for most cases.
- *Balloons:* cutting/scoring balloon – Flextome™ or AngioSculpt™.

Access

- Femoral access is preferred as it provides better guide stability.

Fluoroscopic Views

- LAO-caudal for ostial RCA
- LAO-caudal and AP/LAO-cranial for ostial LM

Steps

- *Lesion preparation:*
  - Ostial lesions tend tends to have higher calcium and fibrous tissue content with increased elastic recoil. Therefore, we prefer to use cutting /scoring balloons prior to deployment of stent.
  - Rotational atherectomy should be considered for heavily calcified lesions.

Fig. 17.1 Placement of an
ostial left main stent in
RAO-cranial view. *Arrow*
marks the proximal edge of
the stent at the ostium

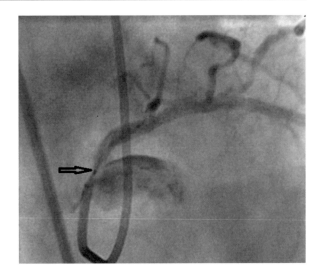

Fig. 17.2 Placement of an
ostial RCA stent in LAO-
caudal view. *Arrow* marks the
proximal edge of the stent at
the ostium

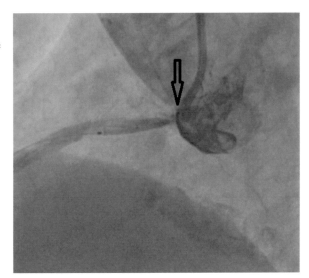

- *Stent positioning*:
  - Since the guide is disengaged during stent positioning, it may be difficult to
    visualize the ostia. If possible, use the presence of ostial calcium to assist with
    stent positioning (Figs. 17.1 and 17.2)
  - *Szabo technique in aorto-ostial lesions*: load the stent onto the primary guide-
    wire in the usual way, then backload the secondary anchor wire (which is
    looped in the aorta) through the most proximal stent strut, and then advance
    the stent into the guide over both the primary guidewire and anchor wire [1].
    Partial flaring of the proximal end of the stent is proposed as a modification to
    facilitate threading of the anchor wire [2].

Fig. 17.3 Use of a Flash
Ostial Balloon™ for
post-dilatation of an ostial
RCA stent. *Arrow* marks the
outer compliant anchoring
(proximal) portion of the
balloon

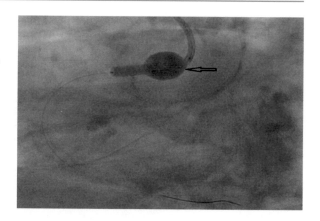

- *Modified Szabo technique in aorto-ostial lesions*: a second wire is placed and
  looped in the aorta to outline the sinus of Valsalva. It defines the junction of
  coronary artery and aorta to assist with stent positioning and also serves to
  provide further guide stability.
- *Stent pull-back technique in branch-ostial lesions*: inflate a balloon at low
  pressure in the parent vessel (size balloon 1:1), then pull back the stent to the
  ostium of the SB to create a dent in the balloon that is positioned in the parent
  vessel [4].
- *Stent deployment:*
  - The stent should be positioned protruding into the aorta by 1–2 mm to prevent
    recoil of the lesion at the stent edge.
  - Avoid using very short (<12 mm) stents to ensure adequate anchoring of the
    stent and to provide adequate lesion coverage distally.
  - Size stent 1:1 ratio and deploy appropriately at high pressures (≥12 atm) to
    ensure optimal apposition.
  - In LM lesions inflation and deflation should be quick (repeat two to three
    times as needed).
  - After stent deployment, we often perform light "flaring" of the ostium of the
    stent.
  - Use of Flash Ostial Balloon™ may be used for flaring of ostial stent (Fig. 17.3).

Complications [3]

- Guide catheter-induced dissection.
- Misplacement of the stent
- Inadequate stent expansion
- Side branch closure
- Stent dislodgment

References

1. Szabo S, Abramowits B, Vaitkuts PT. New technique for aorto-ostial stent placement (Abstr). Am J Cardiol. 2005;96:212 H.
2. Wong P. Two years experience of a simple technique of precise ostial coronary stenting. Catheter Cardiovasc Interv. 2008;72:331–4.
3. Jokhi P, Curzen N. Percutaneous coronary intervention of ostial lesions. EuroIntervention. 2009;5:1–00.
4. Kini A, Moreno P, Steinheimer A. Effectiveness of the stent pull-back technique for nonaorto-ostial coronary narrowings. Am J Cardiol. 2005;96(8):1123–8.

Left Main Coronary Interventions

18

Leslie Innasimuthu, Anitha Rajamanickam,
and Samin Sharma

Interventions of Left main coronary artery (protected and unprotected) require special and careful assessment of other lesions, adequate lesion preparation, and proper
device selection and accurate placement.

Diagnosis of Left Main (LM) Disease

Angiographic diagnosis of LM disease may not be accurate especially in intermediate lesions, especially in short LM lesions and in diffuse disease process. Additional
imaging or physiological assessment is recommended if warranted.

- Role of intravascular ultrasound (IVUS): the cut off for intervention is minimal
  luminal area (MLA) <6 mm². This has been shown to correlate with a fractional
  flow reserve (FFR) <0.8 (Fig. 18.1).
- Role of FFR: FFR values (>0.80) in left main lesions are associated with excellent long-term outcomes. Presence of downstream disease may affect the FFR
  value of LM disease. Myocardial bed supplied by the LM artery may be larger if
  it supplies collaterals to an occluded RCA. It is postulated that the presence of
  significant lesion in either the LAD or the LCX makes the myocardial bed
  smaller for the LM leading to a falsely higher FFR. The left main FFR alone

L. Innasimuthu, MD (✉) • A. Rajamanickam, MD • S. Sharma, MD, FACC
Department of Interventional Cardiology, Mount Sinai Hospital,
One Gustave Levy Place, Madison Avenue, New York 10029, NY, USA
e-mail: antonyleslieuk@gmail.com; arajamanickam@gmail.com,
Anitha.Rajamanickam@mountsinai.org; Samin.sharma@mountsinai.org

© Springer-Verlag London 2014
A. Kini et al. (eds.), *Practical Manual of Interventional Cardiology*,
DOI 10.1007/978-1-4471-6581-1_18

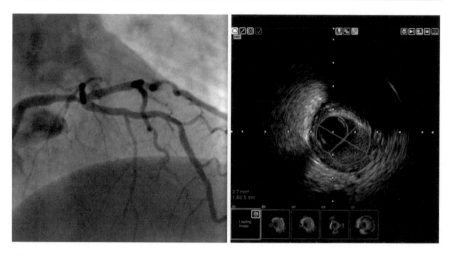

Fig. 18.1 Moderate LM disease by angiography and ivus showed MLA of 3.7 mm²

cannot be accurately measured when there are significant downstream serial lesions. If the LAD and LCX are hemodynamically insignificant, the left main FFR will be accurate.

Protected Versus Unprotected LM Intervention

PCI is preferred approach in protected LM because of high risk associated with repeat CABG. Recent and emerging data have shown that PCI is safe in unprotected LM.

Need for Hemodynamic Support

No hemodynamic support devices are required if LV EF>50 %. We recommend the use of IABP for EF 35–50 % and Impella for EF<20 % and for patients with EF between 20 and 35 %, either IABP or Impella can be used (Fig. 18.2).

Femoral Versus Radial Approach

Both approaches are suitable, but femoral approach is preferred if there is a need for a larger size guide(>6Fr), rotational/orbital atherectomy or hemodynamic support.

Optimal Angiographic Views

AP caudal, AP cranial, LAO cranial, and LAO caudal for visualization of bifurcation

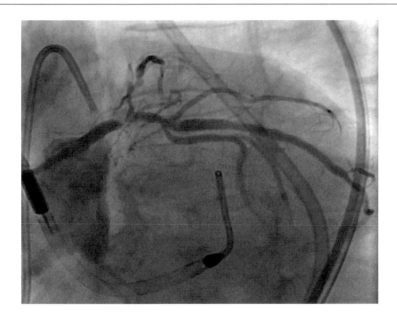

Fig. 18.2 Patient with significant LM disease and LVEF 15%; PCI of LM was performed with Impella support

BMS Versus DES

DES has been shown in multiple trials to have lower MACE event rates as compared to BMS; hence, we recommend DES when feasible.

Approach

Ostial LM

- Sheath size: 6F or 7F
- Guide selection: FL or VL (with side holes). Avoid aggressive guides and deep engagement and ventricularization.
- Wires: Runthrough, Fielder. Buddy wire may be needed to provide additional support.
- Lesion preparation/debulking: predilatation with compliant or semi-compliant balloons. May need Flextome/AngioSculpt for adequate vessel preparation. Rotational atherectomy may be required for heavily calcified lesions (if rotational atherectomy of LM is planned, place a temporary pacing wire). If using rotational atherectomy, disengage the guide slightly and start rota from inside the guide so that the ostium is also adequately prepared.
- Stent selection: DES is preferred

- Stenting strategies
  - Disengage the guide slightly but keep it close enough to enable adequate visualization of the vessel.
    - While holding wires taut, pull back the guide slowly to disengage it from the ostium but while maintaining wire and guide control.
    - Place stent to cover the lesion with a slight overhang into the aorta.
    - Deploy stent with inflation of stent balloon to high pressures at ostium.
    - Postdilate stent and "flare" ostium with high pressure inflation of noncompliant balloon with a portion of the balloon protruding into the aorta.
    - Flash Ostial balloon may be used for flaring of the ostium of the stent.
  - Modified Szabo technique
    - Wire lesion.
    - Place a second, steerable wire in the aorta to stabilize the guide.
    - Place stent over the initial wire and position with 1–2 mm ostial overhang into the aorta.
    - Postdilate with final "flaring" of ostium with noncompliant balloon.

Mid LM

- Sheath size: 6F
- Guide selection: VL vs EBU vs FL
- Wires: Runthrough, Fielder
- Lesion Preparation/Debulking: predilatation with compliant or semi-compliant balloons. May need Flextome/AngioSculpt for moderately calcified vessels and rotational atherectomy may be required for moderate to severely calcified lesions (temporary pacing wire may be needed if rotational atherectomy is planned).
- Stent selection: DES is preferred.
- Stenting strategies: true mid LM lesions have landing zones proximally and distally and hence a focal stent placement after adequate preparation of the lesion is feasible. Postdilate to high pressures using a noncompliant balloon.

Distal LM

- Provisional vs 2-stent strategy: depends on the type of bifurcation lesion and the extent of disease in side branch. If both LAD and LCx ostia have significant disease, 2-stent strategy is preferred otherwise provisional stent strategy is reasonable.
- Sheath size: 7F or 8F
- Guide Selection: VL vs EBU
- Wires: Runthrough, Fielder. Wire both the LAD and LCx and wire the more significant or tighter lesion first. If rotational atherectomy is considered, wire

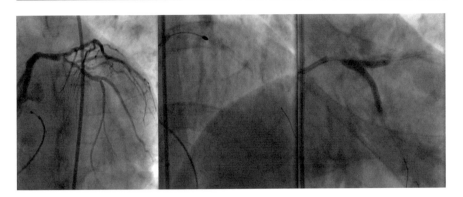

Fig. 18.3   Distal LM disease being debulked by rotational atherectomy

only the vessel which is heavily calcified either directly with a RotaWire or exchange with a Fielder wire/ Finecross microcatheter.
- Lesion preparation/debulking: predilation with compliant or semi-compliant balloons. May need Flextome/AngioSculpt for moderately calcified vessels and rotational atherectomy may be required for moderate to severely calcified lesions (Fig. 18.3). Temporary pacing wire may be needed if rotational atherectomy is planned.
- Stent selection: DES is preferred.
- Stenting strategies:
  - Provisional stenting: if no significant disease in side branch
    - Wire the MBV with Runthrough and the SBV with Fielder.
    - Adequate lesion preparation and debulking should be performed.
    - Confirm position of stent in MBV and deploy.
    - Withdraw SBV wire and rewire SBV through MBV stent strut.
    - Final kissing balloon inflation (KBI)
  - 2-stent strategy (for detailed description of 2-stent strategies, see Chap. 16). Most commonly used 2-stent strategy is SKS or V stenting secondary to the relative ease of procedure and good angiographic results obtained with little hemodynamic disruption also, the need to rewire the side branch is eliminated. If the bifurcation lesion is Medina [0,1,1], then the best strategy would be V stenting strategy. For SKS, PMV must be large enough and at least 2/3 the size of (DMV+SBV).

SKS/V stent

- SKS: >2 mm overlap in LM, V stent: ≤2 mm overlap in LM.
- Wire the MBV with the Runthrough wire and wire SBV with the Fielder wire.

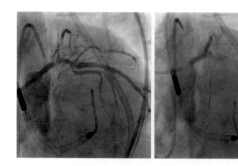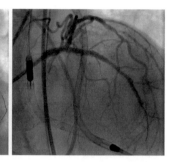

Fig. 18.4 SKS stenting of LM disease with Impella support

- Lesion preparation and debulking should be performed as necessary.
- Both stents positioned with proximal overlap with both markers exactly aligned.
- Simultaneous stent deployment in MBV and SBV (equal pressures) with careful deployment to avoid risk of proximal vessel dissection.
- Final kissing balloon inflation (KBI) (Fig. 18.4).

If the LM is not big enough to take 2 stents and the lesion is Medina type 1, 1, 1, then modified T-stenting strategy could be performed.

Modified T-stenting/Mini Crush

- Wire the MBV with the Runthrough wire and wire SBV with the Fielder wire.
- Lesion preparation as needed.
- Place SBV stent with ≤ 2 mm mm protrusion into the MBV.
- Deploy SBV stent, and then remove wire and stent balloon.
- Deploy MBV stent (completely cover and crush protruding SBV stent).
- Rewire SBV stent through struts of MBV stent and advance a noncompliant balloon (if difficulty is encountered, use a compliant balloon first) to dilate the ostium adequately.
- Final KBI

Less commonly used strategies are DK-CRUSH and culotte technique

Double Kissing CRUSH (DK-CRUSH)

- Wire the MBV with the Runthrough wire and wire SBV with the Fielder wire.
- Adequately prepare and stent the SBV first.
- Balloon the MBV with a noncompliant balloon (First Crush).
- Perform first KBI.
- Take the SBV wire out.
- Stent the MBV (Second Crush).

- Rewire the SB through MV stent struts.
- Perform second KBI.

Culotte stenting

- Wire the MBV with the Runthrough wire and wire SBV with the Fielder wire.
- Lesion preparation and debulking should be performed as necessary.
- Place and deploy SBV stent with the proximal end extending into the PMV for 3–5 mm.
- Remove the jailed wire and rewire the DMV through the SBV stent struts.
- Advance balloon over wire and dilate to open the stent cell in preparation for stenting the MBV.
- Remove the SBV wire.
- Advance the MBV stent and position it to overlap the proximal portion of the SBV stent.
- Deploy the stent and rewire the SBV.
- Final KBI

T-stenting and small protrusion (TAP)

- Wire the MBV with the Runthrough wire and wire SBV with the Fielder wire.
- Lesion preparation as needed.
- Place MBV stent.
- Remove the jailed wire from SBV.
- Rewire the SBV through the MV stent struts.
- Place SBV stent with 1–2 mm protrusion into the MBV.
- Advance balloon in the MBV.
- Deploy the stent in SBV.
- Pull the stent balloon system back and align it with MV balloon and inflate both the balloons simultaneously (Fig. 18.5).

Trifurcation of distal LM   If the distal LM trifurcates into LAD, LCX, and ramus, the treatment of trifurcation lesion could be treated as bifurcation lesion with LM and two larger branches of the three, and leave the smaller of the three branches alone.

Imaging after stent placement   IVUS or OCT can be used to assess adequate stent expansion, complete stent strut apposition, and to rule out any dissections.

Antiplatelet selection   DAPT is recommended at least for 1 year.

Surveillance angiography   There is no evidence for routine use of surveillance angiography, and hence, we recommend for repeat angiography only if clinically indicated.

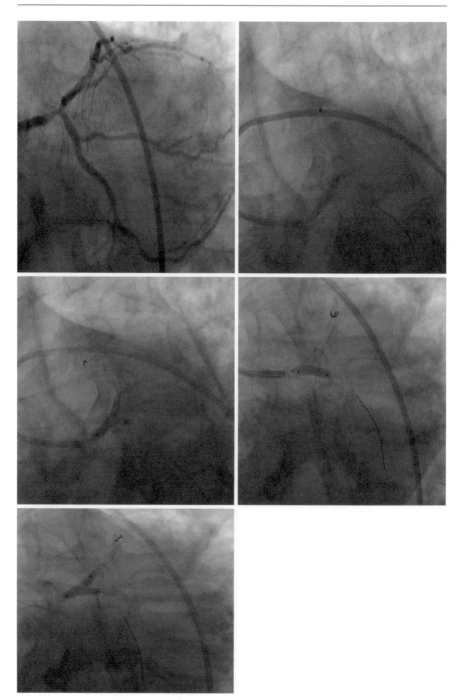

Fig. 18.5 Tap technique for distal LM disease

References

1. Stewart JT, Ward DE, Davies MJ, Pepper JR. Isolated coronary ostial stenosis: observations on the pathology. Eur Heart J. 1987;8:917–20.
2. Sano K, Mintz GS, Carlier SG, et al. Assessing intermediate left main coronary lesions using intravascular ultrasound. Am Heart J. 2007;154:983–8.
3. Popma JJ, Brogan 3rd WC, Pichard AD, Satler LF, Kent KM, Mintz GS, Leon MB. Rotational coronary atherectomy of ostial stenoses. Am J Cardiol. 1993;71:436–8.
4. Baber U, Kini AS, Sharma SK. Stenting of complex lesions: an overview. Nat Rev Cardiol. 2010;7(9):485–96.
5. Park SJ, Hong MK, Lee CW, et al. Elective stenting of unprotected left main coronary artery stenosis: effect of debulking before stenting and intravascular ultrasound guidance. J Am Coll Cardiol. 2001;38:1054–60.
6. Chieffo A, Stankovic G, Bonizzoni E, et al. Early and midterm results of drug-eluting tent implantation in unprotected left main. Circulation. 2005;111:791–5.
7. Sheiban I, Meliga E, Moretti C, et al. Sirolimus-eluting stents vs. bare metal stents for the treatment of unprotected left main coronary artery stenosis. EuroIntervention. 2006;2:356–62.
8. Wood F, Bazemore E, Schneider JE, Jobe RL, Mann T. Technique of left main stenting is dependent on lesion location and distal branch protection. Catheter Cardiovasc Interv. 2005;65:499–503.
9. Melikian N, Airoldi F, Di Mario C. Coronary bifurcation stenting. Current techniques, outcome and possible future developments. Minerva Cardioangiol. 2004;52:365–78.
10. Sharma SK, Choudhury A, Lee J, Kim MC, Fisher E, Steinheimer AM, Kini AS. Simultaneous kissing stents (SKS) technique for treating bifurcation lesions in medium-to-large size coronary arteries. Am J Cardiol. 2004;94(7):913–7.

Chronic Total Occlusions

19

Nagendra Boopathy Senguttuvan, Ravinder Singh Rao, and Annapoorna Kini

Chronic total occlusion (CTO) is defined as a total occlusion with either known duration of more than 3 months or presence of bridging collaterals. CTO has certain favorable and unfavorable characteristics which should be looked for in detail during angiography.

Favorable Characteristics

- Short segment
- Tapered tip
- No side branches or bridging collaterals
- Straight segment
- Functional CTO (faint channel visualized present)

Unfavorable Characteristics

- Calcification (strongest correlation with failure)
- Long segment (>20 mm)
- Blunt stump
- Flush ostial CTO

N.B. Senguttuvan, MD, DM • R.S. Rao, MD • A. Kini, MD, MRCP, FACC (✉)
Department of Interventional Cardiology, Mount Sinai Hospital,
One Gustave Levy Place, Madison Avenue, New York, NY 10029, USA
e-mail: drsnboopathy@gmail.com; drravindersinghrao@yahoo.co.in;
Annapoorna.kini@mountsinai.org

© Springer-Verlag London 2014
A. Kini et al. (eds.), *Practical Manual of Interventional Cardiology*,
DOI 10.1007/978-1-4471-6581-1_19

- Bridging collaterals
- Side branches
- Post CABG/CKD/DM
- LCX CTO

Access

- Single femoral access or radial access if no collaterals are seen from the contralateral vessel
- Dual femoral access
- Femoral and a radial access
- Dual radial access

Approach

- First attempt – antegrade
- Second attempt – antegrade
- Third attempt – retrograde
- Primary retrograde approach can be used for following situations:
  - Ostial CTO
  - Prior failed antegrade approach

Sheath

- 6Fr 45 cm sheath to provide support and overcome tortuosity and 5Fr sheath for retrograde vessel angiogram (femoral access).
- For retrograde CTO attempt, bilateral 6 F 45 cm sheath should be used.

Guides

Selection of guide support is an important step in CTO interventions. It depends on vessel origin, tortuosity, size of aortic root, site of CTO in vessel segment, and experience of the operator (see Table 19.1).

Guide support depends on coaxial alignment and stability of the guide. It can be obtained by three techniques:

- *Mother–child technique*: Use of GuideLiner as a guide extension into coronaries. GuideLiner is advanced into the coronaries over a balloon either deflated or inflated.
- *Balloon anchoring:* Inflate small compliant balloon in a side branch which is not a source of collateral supply.

Table 19.1   Guide selection for CTO

CTO vessel	Guide
Left main CTO – ostial	FL
LAD ostial with long left main	VL
LAD ostial with very short LM/separate origin of LAD	FCL/FL
LAD proximal and mid segment CTO	VL (most commonly used)
LCX	VL (most commonly used)
RCA ostial	JR – side holes
RCA proximal – downsloping with curves	AR2/AL0.75
RCA downsloping – straight	MP
RCA upsloping	IM (most commonly used)
RCA upsloping (Shepherd's Crook)	SCR

Wires

Selection of guidewire is the most important step in the process of opening a CTO (see Fig. 19.1). The wiring techniques used for cap penetration are penetration and drilling.

Wire selection is guided by following characteristics of CTO:

- Presence of micro-channels
- Calcification
- Dissection
- Type of proximal cap: blunt or tapered

CTO with Micro-channels   Hydrophilic wires should be the first choice:

- Fielder™
- Fielder XT™: 0.014 wire which tapers to 0.009

Calcification

- Wires with more penetration power and tip load are used in such cases.
- Wires can be escalated depending on the operator experience and center protocol.
- Wiring technique for proximal cap penetration in such lesions is drilling and penetration. Following escalation sequence is recommended:
  - Miracle 6™.
  - Miracle 9™: Miracle series are good wire for drilling into proximal cap.
  - Confianza Pro 9™.
  - Confianza Pro12™: Confianza wires are good for penetration of proximal cap.
  - Progress™ wires: 0.014 wire tapering to 0.009.

Appearance of CTO	First Choice	Second Choice	Third Choice
Tapered Stump 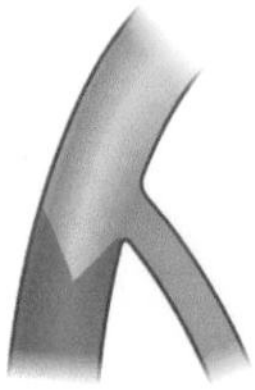	Fielder Fielder XT	Miracle Bro 6	Confienza Pro 9 Confienza Pro 12
Blunt Stump 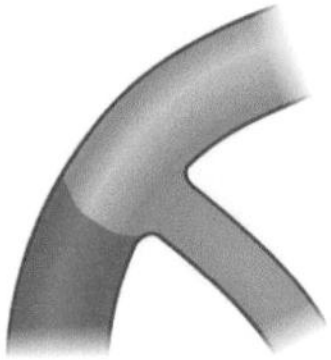	Miracle Bro 6	Confienza Pro 9 Confienza Pro 12	Progress 140 Progress 200
Functional CTO 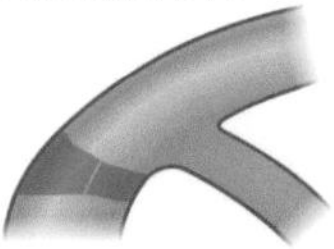	Fielder Fielder XT	Miracle Bro 6	Confienza Pro 9 Confienza Pro 12
Bridging collaterals 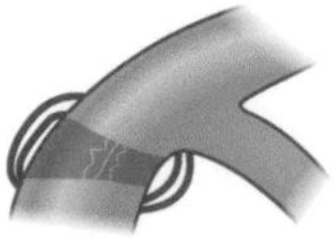	Fielder Fielder XT	Confienza Pro 9 Confienza Pro 12	Progress 200
Severe calcification 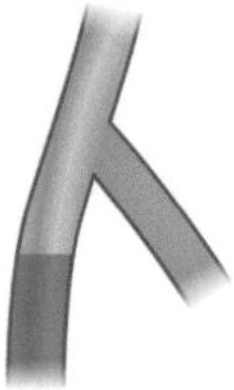	Miracle Bro 6	Progress 200	Confienza Pro 9 Confienza Pro 12

Fig. 19.1 Wire choices based on CTO angiographic features

Tips and Tricks for CTO Wiring

- Single 45–60° bend within 1 cm of tip.
- Tactile feedback from the tip should be continuously assessed by the operator. It is better with hydrophobic wires. Hydrophilic or polymer-coated wires tend to go into subintimal track because of poor feedback.
- Observe and monitor the movement of tip. Suspect it going outside the lumen into pericardium if it moves too freely or into subintimal tissue if restricted.

- Contralateral injection to look at the position of tip.
- Different views to confirm the position of wire with respect to true lumen.
- Wire movement should be 180° back and forth. 360 rotations should be avoided as the wire tip can get embedded into myocardium and break.

Use of Microcatheters

- Finecross™
- Supercross™/Venture catheter™: If CTO is at a bend in a vessel
- Corsair: To cross the lesion if Finecross is not tracking

Traversing the CTO Length

- Once the wire crosses the proximal cap, advance the wire by rotating it 180° back and forth.
- Monitor the movement of wire tip.
- If the wire buckles, it should be retracted, reoriented, and rotated rather than forced through a lesion.
- Use landmarks such as a prior stent or calcification as a guide to wiring.
- Contralateral injection to monitor the advancement.
- To avoid going into the intima, try to wire on the inside portion of any curves, and if in the intima, pull back to where entry into the subintimal space occurred and reposition to enter the main lumen.

Parallel wire technique In the parallel wire technique, if the first wire enters the subintimal space, it is left there, both to mark the channel and to occlude it, and second wires are used to cross the lesion. This technique can also be used with two microcatheters, allowing for easy exchange of the two wires (seesaw technique).

After crossing

- Once the CTO is crossed antegradely, confirm the position of the wire in true lumen by contralateral injection. Injection via Finecross is not advised because it may extend dissection.
- Advance Finecross in the distal vessel and exchange CTO wire for 300 cm Grandslam or a workhorse wire.

Finecross not crossing Following techniques can be used if Finecross is not crossing the lesion:

- Exchange for Corsair. Advance Corsair by torquing movement.
- Smallest profile balloon (1.25/6 mm) and dilatation of CTO segment.
- Rotational atherectomy using 1.25 mm burr. Finecross is abutted to the lesion and wire exchanged for Rota floppy wire. Rotational atherectomy done. Finecross advanced over the wire across the lesion or workhorse wire used side by side the Rotawire.

Removal of microcatheter over a 180/190 cm wire Various techniques are used, but recommended techniques are as follows:

- Exchange for a 300 cm wire and remove Finecross.
- Use of dock extension wire.
- Balloon anchoring (2.5/12 at 12 atm for 6 F guide) of wire inside the guide, once Finecross is pulled proximally. Balloon is advanced into the guide not on the wire, but side by side. Inflated balloon anchors the wire and Finecross is pulled out.

Retrograde Approach

When the CTO cannot be crossed by an antegrade approach, the next option is a retrograde approach.

Selection of collaterals

- There are two types of collaterals – epicardial and septal. Septal channels are the safest and should always be tried first. Septal tortuosity and not the size can be a limiting factor in wire placement. Epicardial channels often have a corkscrew anatomy making them more difficult; however it can still be used to advance a microcatheter through it.

Retrograde CTO steps

- *Step 1: Septal collateral wiring*. Selection of suitable septal collaterals: Any septal collateral that is less tortuous can be selected. Usually septals are profiled better in RAO view with slight cranial or caudal projections.
    - Profile the septal collaterals.
    - Enter the septal artery with Fielder FC, Whisper, or Fielder with Corsair catheter (150 cm) (see Fig. 19.2).
    - Surf the septals and slowly advance the wire with each heart beat into the distal epicardial vessel.
- *Step 2: Crossing the distal cap, traversing the length, and crossing proximal cap*:
    - Attempt with Fielder wire.
    - Escalate to Miracle™ and Confianza™ wires as judged by the operator (Fig. 19.3).
- *Step 3: Externalizing the wire*:
    - Advance the wire into antegrade guide (Fig. 19.4).
    - Trap the wire with 2.5/12 balloon in the antegrade guide (Fig. 19.5).
    - Advance Corsair over the wire into the antegrade guide.
    - Exchange the wire for 335 cm 0.014 Viper wire and externalize the wire out of the guide. Remove copilot from the guide. Insert wire introducer in the copilot. Thread the wire into the introducer and then attach copilot to the guide (Fig. 19.6).

Fig. 19.2 *Red arrow*:
Fielder FC wire used for
surfing the septal collaterals
and seen entering into distal
vessel. *Blue arrow*: Corsair
catheter

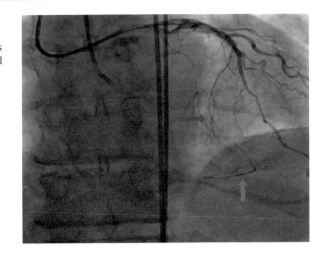

Fig. 19.3 Fielder wire™
escalated to Confianza Pro™
12 with short tip and distal
and proximal caps crossed

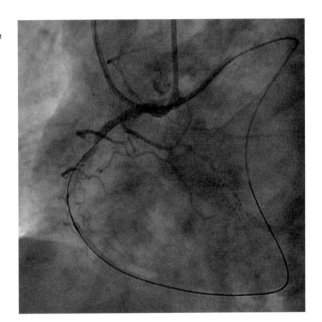

- *Step 4: Kissing microcatheter technique*:
  - Advance Finecross antegradely over the externalized wire.
  - Pull back Corsair and advance Finecross antegradely, distally in the CTO vessel.
  - Approximate both the microcatheters in distal vessel.
  - Remove the Viper wire. This technique prevents "cheese-grating" phenomenon and retrograde vessel dissection (Fig. 19.7).

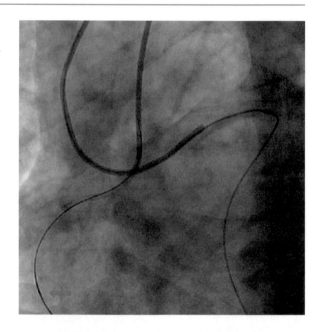

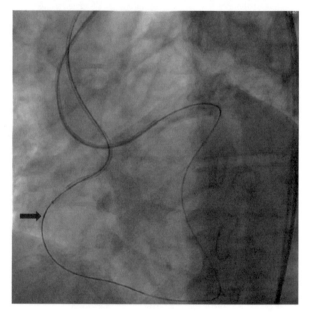

Fig. 19.4 Wire advanced into the antegrade guide catheter. *Red arrow*: Corsair catheter

Fig. 19.5 *Red arrow*: 2.5/12 balloon used for trapping the wire in guide. *Green arrow*: GuideLiner used as guide extension in difficult cases were Corsair cannot be advanced into the antegrade guide. *Blue arrow*: Corsair catheter

Fig. 19.6 Corsair (*red arrow*) advanced into the antegrade catheter. Retrograde wire removed and exchanged for a 330 cm Viper wire which is externalized from the copilot of antegrade guide

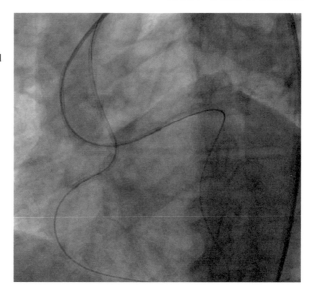

Fig. 19.7 Kissing microcatheter technique (KMT): Finecross (*red arrow*) is advanced antegradely over the externalized Viper wire into the distal vessel. Simultaneously, Corsair (*blue arrow*) is withdrawn into the distal vessel where both Corsair and Finecross approximate each other. Viper wire is removed along with Corsair catheter. This technique prevents cheese-grating phenomenon and protects retrograde vessel from guide-catheter-induced dissection

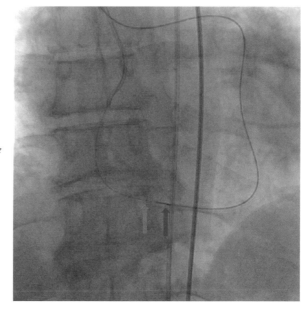

Fig. 19.8 300 cm
Grandslam™ wire is
advanced into the distal
vessel. Finecross removed.
Predilatation done. Stent
placed and successful
intervention of RCA CTO
completed

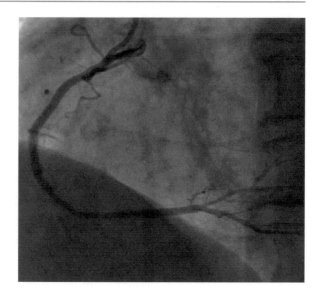

- *Step: 5 Removal of Corsair*:
    - Remove Corsair. Look for deep engagement of the retrograde guide. Always do retrograde vessel angiogram, looking for any dissection and thrombus.
    - Retrograde guide can be removed.
- *Step 6: Opening the CTO*:
    - 300 cm Grandslam wire is advanced into the distal vessel. Finecross removed (Fig. 19.8).
    - Open CTO antegradely.
    - Final angiogram to rule out any perforation, dissection, or other cath-related complications.

Other Techniques

- CART (controlled antegrade retrograde tracking and reentry)
- Reverse CART
- STAR (subintimal tracking and reentry)

When to Stop CTO Procedure

- Fluoro time >60 min, if CTO is not crossed
- AK > 5 Gy, if CTO is not crossed
- Patient or operator fatigue
- Perforation, dissection, or other coronary complication limiting further procedure
- Large volume of contrast used

ACS: STEMI/Non-STEMI Intervention

20

Rahul Sawant, Anitha Rajamanickam, and Joseph Sweeny

Acute Coronay Syndrome

Acute coronary syndrome is a spectrum ranging from ST elevation myocardial infarction to troponin-negative unstable angina. Plaque rupture or erosion leads to thrombus formation resulting in ischemic myocardial damage. Guidelines recommend primary angioplasty for patients with STEMI and early invasive strategy [<72 h] for patients with high risk ACS.

Tips for the management of patients with acute coronary syndrome:

1. Keep it simple. Avoid bifurcation stenting due to risk of higher of stent thrombosis.
2. Ensure the lesion is adequately covered by the stent, use longer stents in thrombotic lesions.
3. Treat the infarct-related artery only. Do not treat nonculprit lesion unless cardiogenic shock or severe flow limiting stenosis distal to the culprit lesion is present.
4. Minimize contrast use.

Non-STEMI

Pharmacological therapy prior to invasive therapy

R. Sawant, MD (✉) • A. Rajamanickam, MD • J. Sweeny, MD
Department of Interventional Cardiology, Mount Sinai Hospital,
One Gustave Levy Place, Madison Avenue, New York 10029, NY, USA
e-mail: drrahulsawant@hotmail.com; arajamanickam@gmail.com,
Anitha.Rajamanickam@mountsinai.org; Joseph.sweeny@mountsinai.org

© Springer-Verlag London 2014   187
A. Kini et al. (eds.), *Practical Manual of Interventional Cardiology*,
DOI 10.1007/978-1-4471-6581-1_20

Dual antiplatelet therapy

ASA 162–325 mg plus
P2Y12 inhibitor [one of the following]:
- Clopidogrel: 600 mg loading dose (300 mg if increased risk of bleeding) followed by 75 mg daily.
- Prasugrel: 60 mg loading dose, followed by 10 mg daily if weight >100 kg and 5 mg if weight <100 kg. It is contraindicated in patients with prior CVA, weight <60 kg, and age >75 years.
- Ticagrelor: 180 mg loading dose followed by 90 mg twice daily.

Anticoagulation [one of the following]

- Bivalirudin 0.75 mg/kg and then infusion of 1.75 mg/kg/h. If creatinine clearance is <30 ml/min, bolus dose remains the same, but infusion dose is reduced to 1 mg/kg/h or 0.25 mg/kg/h if on dialysis.
- Unfractionated heparin: 70 units/kg up to 4,000 units followed by 12 units/kg infusion up to 1,000 units. Target ACT 300 s.

Adjunctive medical therapy

- Nitrates (sublingual/intravenous/transdermal) helps in relieving pain. It is contraindicated if systolic BP < 100 mmHg or if there is right ventricular infarction or recent use of sidenafilvardenafil(<24 hrs) or tadalafil (<48 hrs).
- Beta-blockers (Oral/IV). It is contraindicated in patients who are at the risk of developing cardiogenic shock [age > 70, Killip class 3 or 4, or systolic BP <120 mmHg].
- High-dose statins (within first 24 h) for its pleiotropic effect.
- ACE inhibitors (within first 24 h), especially in patients with systolic LV dysfunction and used with caution in patients with relative hypotension.

Bare metal stent (BMS) or drug eluting stent (DES)

- Lower rate of major adverse cardiovascular events with DES is solely driven by lower rate of target vessel revascularization.
- Safety and efficacy of DES in unstable coronary syndrome is similar to stable coronary disease (elective PCI).
- Higher rate of restenosis with BMS.
- BMS preferable if concerns about compliance, affordability, bleeding history, or impending operations which cannot be postponed for a year.

Duration of dual antiplatelet therapy post PCI

- ASA 81–162 mg daily lifelong for both BMS and DES.
- Clopidogrel/prasugrel/ticagrelor for at least 1 month if BMS. Ideally for 12 months post ACS.
- Clopidogrel/prasugrel/ticagrelor for 12 months if DES.

STEMI

Dual antiplatelet therapy   ASA 162–325 mg plus one of the P2Y12 inhibitors as noted above [non-STEMI]

Anticoagulation   Bivalirudin IV bolus and infusion is routinely used for coronary intervention in catheter lab. IV 5,000 units of heparin at the first contact in ER may be administered.

Diagnostic angiogram

If ST segment elevation on ECG suggests LCA obstruction:
- Obtain femoral artery access, assess opening pressure, and give bolus dose of bivalirudin.
- Advance JR4 diagnostic catheter into LV to measure LVEDP. IV furosemide if LVEDP >20 mm of Hg is given after finishing PCI.
- Perform manual injection ventriculogram to assess LV function (limit dye use).
- Perform single injection of RCA in LAO cranial view (15 LAO, 30 Cranial) and pan for late filling.
- To evaluate LCA, engage with VL3.5 guide catheter and take AP caudal and AP cranial projections to assess for lesion location.

If ST segment elevation on ECG suggests RCA obstruction (Fig. 20.1):
- If there is any electric instability or conduction delay or bradycardia, insert temporary pacing wire.
- Take 2 views of LCA with JL4 catheter (AP caudal and AP cranial).
- Advance IM/FR4 guide catheter (with side holes) into LV to assess LVEDP.
- Inject RCA using minimal dye.
- If borderline BP (SBP <100 mm of Hg, HR >90 beats/min, or LVEDP >25 mm of Hg) consider IABP insertion on contralateral groin and IV furosemide at the end of primary PCI.

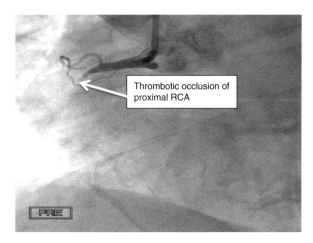

Thrombotic occlusion of proximal RCA

Fig. 20.1 Thrombotic occlusion of proximal RCA

Fig. 20.2 Thrombotic plaque in mid RCA

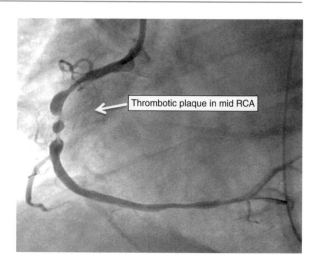

Thrombotic plaque in mid RCA

- If patient presents with signs of cardiogenic shock (SBP <90 mm of Hg, HR>110 beats/min), consider IABP or Impella at the start of the case.

Coronary intervention

- Check ACT to ensure adequate anticoagulation (goal >300).
- Wire with workhorse wire with a soft tip such as Runthrough™ or BMW Universal™ to cross occlusive thrombotic lesion in order to reduce the risk of dissection (Fig. 20.2). Use balloon support with a 2×15 mm compliant balloon.
- Once the lesion is crossed by the wire, advance balloon across the lesion to break up the thrombus (dottering).
- Take cine angiographic picture to document restoration of distal vessel flow and document distal wire position.
- Look for distal embolization.
- If significant thrombus is visualized in the lesion, consider aspiration catheter like Pronto™ or Export™ (Fig. 20.3). In the presence of extensive thrombus burden (grade≥to 4) is evident, then mechanical thrombectomy device like AngioJet™ may be beneficial.
- Stenting: We attempt to direct stent without predilatation (Fig. 20.4). Predilatation can lead to distal embolization of the thrombus. If the stent is unable to cross the lesion, predilatation should be performed with a small compliant balloon (2–2.5 mm diameter and 12–15 mm length at 8–10 atm). For same reasons, one should try to avoid postdilatation. However, if the stent does not fully expand, postdilate the stent with a 1:1 high pressure balloon at no more than 16 atm.

Fig. 20.3 Pronto™
[aspiration catheter] in mid
RCA

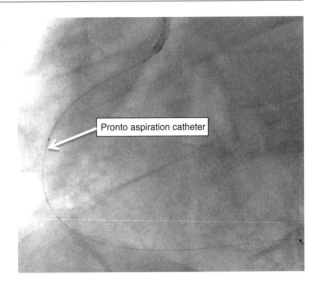

Pronto aspiration catheter

Fig. 20.4 DES deployed in
proximal/mid RCA

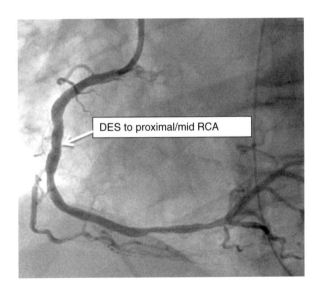

DES to proximal/mid RCA

Treatment of distal embolization/slow reflow/no reflow

- Medication to treat distal embolization and slow flow/no reflow in an infarct-related artery can be administered through the guide catheter or through a special delivery catheter which can be delivered to the target vessel using 0.014″ wire.
- Twin-Pass Catheter™: Allows the operator to deliver medication through the OTW lumen while leaving the original treatment lumen in place.

If Twin-Pass Catheter™ is not available, medication can be delivered through the aspiration lumen of Pronto™ or Export™ catheter. If this catheter has been used for thrombus suction, make sure that lumen has been flushed thoroughly to remove any residual clot.

Medication used to treat distal embolization

- Verapamil 250 µg bolus max 2,000 µg (vasodilator)
- Adenosine 10–20 µg bolus (vasodilator)
- Sodium nitroprusside 50–200 µg, max 1,000 µg (direct NO donor)

Coronary Artery Bypass Graft Interventions

21

Anitha Rajamanickam and Samin Sharma

Ten-year patency rates are around 90 % for internal mammary arteries [IMA] and 57 % for saphenous veins grafts [SVG] [1]. Redo-CABG has been shown to have reduced graft patency rates, incomplete symptom relief and very high mortality at 11 %, 25 % and 39 % for first, second and third re-operations, respectively, as compared to 4 % mortality rates for the first CABG [2, 3]. PCI is increasingly preferred in symptomatic patients with graft vessel disease [4] and PCI of native vessel, if feasible, is preferred over PCI of the grafts [4].

SVG Interventions

Restenosis rates after SVG stenting are approximately 25–30 % at 1 year after BMS and 8–10 % after DES [4–6]. Success is less likely in grafts >3 years old and aorto-ostial lesions which are more prone to distal embolization as well. PCI of CTO (>3 months) of SVGs in a symptomatic patient should not be considered unless there is an antegrade channel present and there is no possibility of native vessel PCI. [class III ACC/AHA recommendation].

Equipment

- *Sheath*: 6 Fr long sheath
- *Guide catheter*:
  - For left-sided bypass grafts – AR2, IM, AL 0.75, AL1, or AL 2
  - For right-sided bypass grafts – MP1, AR2, AL 0.75 or AL 1

A. Rajamanickam, MD (✉) • S. Sharma, MD, FACC
Department of Interventional Cardiology, Mount Sinai Hospital,
One Gustave Levy Place, Madison Avenue, New York 10029, NY, USA
e-mail: arajamanickam@gmail.com, Anitha.Rajamanickam@mountsinai.org;
Samin.sharma@mountsinai.org

© Springer-Verlag London 2014
A. Kini et al. (eds.), *Practical Manual of Interventional Cardiology*,
DOI 10.1007/978-1-4471-6581-1_21

- *Wires*: Runthrough or FilterWire for SVGs if technically feasible.
- *Balloon/stent*: Size the balloons and stents no larger than the reference diameter. Balloon catheters with extra-long (145-cm) shafts may be needed.

Access Femoral or radial

Fluoroscopic Views Initial view is straight LAO

- RAO caudal or AP caudal for graft to LCX or OM
- RAO cranial or AP cranial for graft to LAD or diagonal
- LAO cranial or AP cranial for graft to RPDA

Steps

- Coaxial engagement.
- Intra-graft verapamil, nitroprusside, nicardipine, or adenosine to prevent no-reflow phenomenon.
- Wire the lesion with 0.014″ wire.
- Embolic protection device (EPD) is a class I indication during SVG PCI to prevent distal embolization. Assess the distal landing zone to decide on the type of EPD (see Chap. 10 Basics of Intracoronary devices for types and steps of EPD use).
- Primary stenting is preferred for all SVG interventions if possible to minimize distal embolization.
- If there is difficulty encountered in advancing the stent across the lesion then perform the following steps.
  - Advance the stent while the patient performs deep breathing maneuvers.
  - Use a small 2.0 to 2.5 / 12 to 15 mm compliant balloon to predialte the lesion
  - Use the buddy wire technique but ensure that the stent is deployed over the EPD wire and the buddy wire is removed before the stent is deployed.
  - If all the above techniques fail, consider using a Guideliner with extreme caution over the EPD wire.

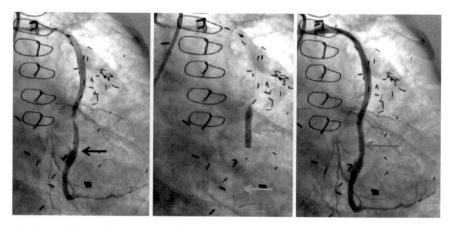

Fig. 21.1 SVG to LPL intervention. *Black arrow*: 90 % stenosis at mid SVG to LPL, *green arrow*: Spider Filter. *Blue arrow*: angioplasty with 3.0/18 noncomplaint balloon, *red arrow*: deployment of DES [3.5/20]

- Never oversize the balloon or stent.
- Stent from "normal" segment to "normal" segment (Fig. 21.1).
- Avoid high pressure (>12-14 atm) or postdilation.

Complications

- No-reflow: etiology is complex but mainly caused by distal embolization of thrombotic material. Delivery of nitroprusside or verapamil to the distal vessels using a Twinpass micro-catheter or EPD use may help prevent this phenomenon. (see Chap. 23: Coronary Complications: Diagnosis and Treatment).
- Perforation: prevention of perforation by ensuring guidewire is intraluminal, not inflating a balloon in a subintimal location and avoiding overexpansion of the graft.

Arterial Graft Interventions

LIMA patency rates are high, around 90–95 % at 10 years [1]. PCI of the LIMA or through the LIMA has a high success rate. There is a low incidence of abrupt closure, distal embolization, acute myocardial infarction, or emergency coronary artery bypass graft surgery. Usually failure of PCI is due to the inherent technical challenges due to inability to navigate the tortuosity to reach the lesion.

Equipment

- *Sheath:* 6 Fr Long sheath
- *Guide catheter:* use shorter guides to access distal lesions though long tortuous grafts.
  - LIMA: IM 90 cm (Fig. 21.2).
  - RIMA: 3DRC or no-torque (Fig. 21.3).

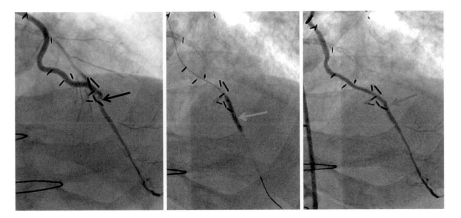

Fig. 21.2 LIMA intervention. *Black arrow*: 90 % stenosis at site of LIMA anastomosis to distal LAD. *Blue arrow*: angioplasty with 2.0/15 noncomplaint balloon. *Red arrow*: deployment of DES [2.5/18]

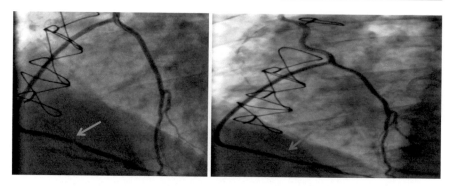

Fig. 21.3 RIMA graft intervention. *Black arrow*: 90 % stenosis RPDA limb of the RIMA Y graft. *Red arrow*: post direct DES stent deployment [3.0/15]

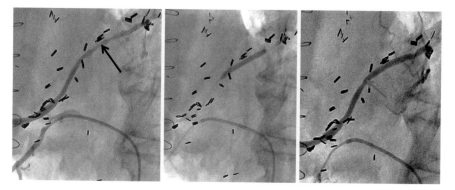

Fig. 21.4 Gastroepiploic graft intervention. *Black arrow*: 70 % stenosis of mid gastroepiploic graft to distal LPL. *Blue arrow*: direct stenting with DES [3.5/33]. *Red arrow*: post stent deployment

- Free radial: usually AR2 for left-sided grafts and MP1 for right-sided grafts will suffice.
- Gastroepiploic: engage with cobra diagnostic catheter and wire the lesion with a 300 cm wire and exchange for an FR guide ± use of a GuideLiner (Fig. 21.4).
- *Wires:*
  - Fielder or other hydrophilic wires and nitinol core guidewires are more flexible and unlikely to kink or straighten the IMA and less likely to cause pseudostenosis. In rare cases, extrasupport guidewires such as mailman may be required.
- *Balloon:*
  - Size the balloons and stents no larger than the reference diameter.
  - Use longer shaft balloons and stents if needed.

Access

- LIMA: femoral/left radial for LIMA
- RIMA: femoral/right radial for RIMA

Fluoroscopic Views

- Initial view for engaging: AP straight
- Ostium of LIMA: AP straight or a 45° to 60° RAO or LOA
- Anastomotic site of LIMA: AP cranial, RAO straight and rarely 90° LAO
- Anastomotic site of RIMA: depends on artery bypassed (see Chap. 2: Perfect Angiographic Views)

Steps

- Engaging may be difficult. The key is to avoid dissection, as this may be disastrous especially if the IMA is the primary vessel perfusing the heart.
- Watch out for spasm when engaging the vessel. Give intracoronary nitroglycerin or verapamil on engagement of IMA.
- Avoid deep guide intubation of the IMA.
- Always monitor the pressure tracing closely.
- Hand inject contrast gently into the IMA to confirm position of the guide and wire the lesion with hydrophilic 0.014″ wire.
- If you have difficulty engaging LIMA:
  - Rule out groin tortuosity. Use a long sheath for access.
  - Use straight 45° to 90° projection to elongate the arch as it helps engage in presence of tortuous subclavian artery.
  - Wire the IMA using a hydrophilic 0.014″ wire with the guide close to the ostium and rail the guide into the IMA ostium with a transit catheter or balloon support (2.0/12 mm) the wire.
  - Use a diagnostic catheter to engage the IMA and exchange for guide over a long 300 cm 0.014″ wire.
- Lower threshold to use GuideLiner for support, microcatheters, and movable and directional tip catheters (Venture or Supracross) to help wiring and stenting.

Complications

- Dissection or perforation of IMA: Always have ready access to a covered stent and surgical backup (see Chap. 10 for Covered Stent Insertion/Chap. 21 for Management).
- Spasm: IC nitro or verapamil.
- Pseudostenosis/According: occurs in redundant tortuous vessels and mimics actual dissection or closure of the IMA vessel. Pull the wire back so that the soft flexible portion of the wire is across the area of interest. The soft distal portion of the wire will conform to the tortuosity and eliminate the pseudostenosis of these vessels but will allow access to the vessel if this is actually a dissection or acute closure.

Special Cases
- *Immediate post-CABG ischemic symptoms* – class I guidelines for PCI – Make sure that the wire is intracoronary and size balloon 0.5:1 to avoid disruption of sutures and postoperative fatal bleeding.

References

1. Sharma S, Makkar RM. Percutaneous intervention on the LIMA: tackling the tortuosity. J Invasive Cardiol. 2003;15(6):359–62. PubMed PMID: 12777679.
2. Hannan EL, Kilburn H, O'Donnell JF, et al. Adult open heart surgery in New York State. JAMA. 1990;264:2768–74.
3. Dohi M, Miyata H, Doi K, Okawa K, Motomura N, Takamoto S, Yaku H; on behalf of the Japan Cardiovascular Surgery Database. The off-pump technique in redo coronary artery bypass grafting reduces mortality and major morbidities: propensity score analysis of data from the Japan Cardiovascular Surgery Database. Eur J Cardiothorac Surg. 2014. [Epub ahead of print] PubMed PMID:24623172.
4. Behboudi F, Vakili H, Hashemi SR, Hekmat M, Safi M, Namazi MH. Immediate results and six-month clinical outcome after percutaneous coronary intervention in patients with prior coronary artery bypass surgery. J Tehran Heart Cent. 2011;6(1):31–6. Epub 2011 Feb 28. PubMed PMID: 23074602; PubMed Central PMCID: PMC3466866.
5. Farooq V, Serruys PW, Zhang Y, Mack M, Ståhle E, Holmes DR, Feldman T, Morice MC, Colombo A, Bourantas CV, de Vries T, Morel MA, Dawkins KD, Kappetein AP, Mohr FW. Short-term and long-term clinical impact of stent thrombosis and graft occlusion in the SYNTAX trial at 5 years: Synergy Between Percutaneous Coronary Intervention with Taxus and Cardiac Surgery trial. J Am Coll Cardiol. 2013;62(25):2360–9. doi:10.1016/j.jacc.2013.07.106. Epub 2013 Oct 16. PubMed PMID: 24140677.
6. Sabik 3rd JF, Lytle BW, Blackstone EH, Houghtaling PL, Cosgrove DM. Comparison of saphenous vein and internal thoracic artery graft patency by coronary system. Ann Thorac Surg. 2005;79(2):544–51; discussion 544–51. PubMed PMID: 15680832.

Calcific Lesion Interventions

22

Anitha Rajamanickam and Samin Sharma

Procedural inability to deploy stents was shown to be more frequent in patients with calcified lesions than in those with noncalcified lesions (8.2 % vs 1.8 %, respectively) [1, 2]. Optimal stent delivery and apposition in these calcified lesions mandate adequate debulking prior to stent deployment.

Currently Available Techniques to Debulk Calcium in Target Lesions

- High-pressure noncomplaint balloons
- Cutting balloons
  - Flextome™
  - AngioSculpt catheter™
- Atherectomy devices:
  - Rotational atherectomy device™ [RA]
  - CSI orbital atherectomy device™ [OA]
  - Excimer laser atherectomy device™ [ELCA]

Though studies have consistently demonstrated procedural success of >95 % and a good safety profile in experienced hands [3], RA is underused (only utilized in 1.2 % of PCI performed in 2011) [4] as the setup is considered cumbersome and the learning curve to get proficient is steep. Orbital atherectomy device is the newly FDA-approved device for treatment of severely calcified coronary lesions. It has an easier setup and a faster learning curve when compared to RA.

A. Rajamanickam, MD (✉) • S. Sharma, MD, FACC
Department of Interventional Cardiology, Mount Sinai Hospital,
One Gustave Levy Place, Madison Avenue, New York 10029, NY, USA
e-mail: arajamanickam@gmail.com, Anitha.Rajamanickam@mountsinai.org;
Samin.sharma@mountsinai.org

© Springer-Verlag London 2014
A. Kini et al. (eds.), *Practical Manual of Interventional Cardiology*,
DOI 10.1007/978-1-4471-6581-1_22

Rotational Atherectomy

Rotational atherectomy (RA) differentially ablates calcified plaques by plaque abrasion with microparticle embolization in order to achieve luminal enlargement. It is particularly valuable in severely calcified lesions [5, 6]. It has also been demonstrated to be safe and efficient in diffuse instent restenosis [7]. High-speed rotational atherectomy with the Rotablator™ devices pulverize fibrotic and inelastic plaque components into microparticles less than 10 μm in size using diamond-coated burrs rotating approximately at 140,000–160,000 revolutions per minute (RPM) (Figs. 22.1 and 22.2). The high-speed rotation minimizes friction and enables the burr to easily navigate through tortuous stenotic vessels. The differential cutting avoids ablation of non-diseased segments proximal and distal to the target lesion. The Rotalink burr catheter is 135 cm long sheath with outer diameter of 4.3 Fr, which protects the arterial tissue from the spinning driveshaft and permits passage of saline to lubricate the driveshaft. The elliptical-shaped brass burr is nickel-coated and has microscopic diamond crystals embedded on the distal edge. The diamond crystals are 20 μm in size with 5 μm extruding from the nickel coating. The proximal surface of the burr is smooth and comes in various sizes (Fig. 22.2).

Rotational Atherectomy Steps

Patient Preparation

- Evaluate for egg allergy.
- Evaluate if the patient is adequately hydrated and is able to receive vasodilators.
- Temporary pacemaker for RCA/dominant LCx.
- Dual antiplatelet therapy on board.
- Anticoagulation with bivalirudin or heparin.

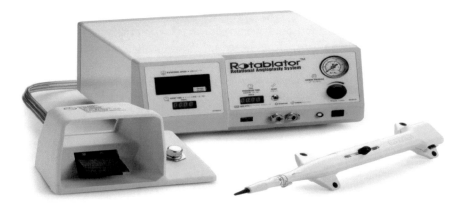

Fig. 22.1 Rotational atherectomy equipment (© 2014 Boston Scientific Corporation or its affiliates. All rights reserved. Used with permission of Boston Scientific Corporation)

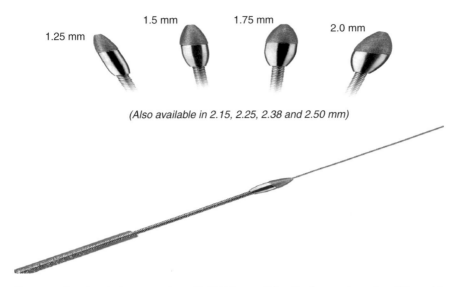

(Also available in 2.15, 2.25, 2.38 and 2.50 mm)

Fig. 22.2 Rotational atherectomy burrs (© 2014 Boston Scientific Corporation or its affiliates. All rights reserved. Used with permission of Boston Scientific Corporation)

Console Preparation

- Connect the Rotaflush fluid (5,000 U of heparin + 5 mg of nitroglycerin + 5 mg of verapamil + rotaglide in 1 L normal saline) with a three-way stopcock to the Rota advancer using a pressure bag to maintain continuous infusion of the flush solution through the Rotablator device.
- Connect tachometer fiberoptic cable to the blue plug named "fiberoptic" located front of the console.
- Connect air cable to the front of console.
- The foot pedal connection (including Dynaglide) is comprised of a pink, a blue and a green cable. Connect the pink cable to the front plug (orange plug) and blue/green cable to the back of the console.
- Connect the nitrogen compressor tank to the back of console. The wheel of the on/off valve on the gas tank is turned on by moving it to the right. Check that the psi is around 90 to 110 (on the wheel which has markings upto 200 psi). The tank valve (on the wheel which has markings upto 4000 psi) should show a psi of at least 500 which is the lowest acceptable range to begin a procedure. A psi of ≥ 750 is preferred as the tank will not run out of nitrogen during the procedure.
- Plug in the power cord and turn on the switch. The light in front of the console will then turn on.
- The front console has a display for event time, procedure time with a reset button, a tachometer, a knob to control the Rotaburr speed, a pressure gauge, and a Dynaglide light indicator.

Equipment

- Burr size: roughly ½ the size of the treatment vessel. If FineCross or a small 1.5 mm balloon crosses the lesion, then start with 1.5 mm burr; otherwise, and in case of CTO, use a 1.25 mm burr. Burrs can be exchanged and upsized to a larger burr if needed.
- Guide catheter: use a 6 Fr catheter if a burr size <1.75 mm, 7Fr catheter for 2.0 burr, and 8Fr catheter for a 2.25 burr.
- Guidewire: the 2 Rotawires used are Rota-Floppy and the Rota Extra Support Guide wires (330 mm, 0.009 inches body with a maximum tip diameter is 0.014 inch). The Rotawire has a long, tapered shaft designed for flexibility and to minimize wire bias. The Extra Support guide wire has a short, tapered shaft that maximizes straightening of the vessel.
- NC balloon: size the balloon to the same size as treatment vessel (1:1).
- The guidewire clip that is packaged with the rotawire needs to be used as a torquer to avoid any kinking or fractures while torquing the wire. It also acts as a secondary brake.
- Carefully remove the distal tip of delicate Rota-floppy wire and wipe generously with a wet 4×4 making only three large loops and set it aside. Take care not to bend or kink the Rotawire.

Initial Procedure Steps

- Direct wiring with Rota-floppy wire is performed in around 30 % of lesions. Otherwise exchange for Rota wires using a Runthrough™ or Fielder™ wire with a FineCross™/1.5 mm balloon support is performed. In heavily calcified lesions the Rota Extrasupport wire may be required.
- Backload and advance the burr over the guidewire to the copilot.
- Place a wire clip at end of Rotawire and reconfirm this verbally.
- Turn on flush solution and perform RPM check with the burr held upright in the air and away from any entanglements [do not touch the burr].
- Activate the Dynaglide mode using the foot button. This is the small round button on the right. A brief tap is all that is required to turn Dynaglide on and off. When Dynaglide mode is switched on, the Dynaglide light on the console turns green.
- Advance the burr though guiding catheter to the ostium of the artery.
- For distal lesions advance the burr manually on Dynaglide mode till the burr is just proximal to the lesion after the steps to remove tension are performed.

Steps to Remove Tension/Inertia from System

- Move advancer knob back and forth.
- Open copilot and move burr back and forth under fluoroscopy.
- Brief Dynaglide tap under fluoroscopy to check for sudden burr advancements, jumps, or residual tension. This speed check is safer when performed at lower speeds. For Dyna tap, tap the square foot pedal on the left once. For Rota runs this needs to be pressed lightly and continuously like a car accelerator as long as the runs last. Once your foot is taken off the pedal the rotaburr turns off.

Rotablation Steps

- Advance the burr slowly with a to-and-fro pecking motion.
- Use short burr run times [15–20 s] and low speeds [140,000–160,000 RPM].
- Avoid significant drops in RPM [>5,000 RPM for >5 s].
- Flush the system during the runs using diluted contrast/saline [Ratio of 1:10].
- Keep SBP > 100 using boluses of IVF or 100 mcg doses of IV Neo-Synephrine if needed. Monitor for reflex bradycardia.
- Total procedure time should not exceed 3 min.

Final Steps

- Remove burr on Dynaglide mode with the break release in the "On" position (depress the black button on the console). Make sure the second operator advances the rota wire at the same speed that the Rota burr is being withdrawn so that the tip of the wire and guide stays in the same position.
- Remove the wire clip and turn off the flush solution and completely remove the burr from wire.
- Take a CINE image to rule out any complications.
- Advance workhorse wire [Fielder™ or Runthrough™] across the lesion parallel to Rotawire™.
- Post-Rota PTCA with NC Balloon [size balloon 1:1 to the true vessel size].
- Position stent and make sure the Rotawire is removed prior to stent deployment.

Complications

- Transient heart block [pacemaker if needed]
- Wire bias
- Dissections (for management see Chap. 21)
- Perforations (for management see Chap. 21)
- Slow flow/no reflow (for management see Chap. 21)
- Transient
- Rota burr entrapment

Burr Entrapment The burr is olive shaped and has diamond coating at its distal surface for antegrade ablation, but no diamonds on the proximal part which prohibits backward ablation. If a burr was advanced beyond a tight calcified lesion or embedded in a long, angulated, and heavily calcified lesion, it can be entrapped. During high-speed rotation, the heat may enlarge the space between plaques and since the coefficient of friction during motion is less than that at rest, the burr may pass the calcified lesion easily without debulking a significant amount of calcified tissue but the burr may get stuck on the way back. This is called the "kokesi" phenomenon.

Prevention of Burr Entrapment

- Gentle pecking motion especially in long, heavily calcified and angulated lesions
- Short runs of Rotablation of less than 20 s.

- Avoid burr speeds of greater than 160,000 RPM.
- RPM should not drop >10 % during burr advancement.
- Maintain continuous high-pressure flushing of Rota burr with Rota flush solution.
- Use stiffer wire if needed when difficulty is encountered during the passage of the burr.

Management of Burr Entrapment

- Never attempt to start the burr if it has stalled in the lesion.
- First try pulling back the Rotablator system by manual traction.
- Intracoronary nitroglycerin and/or verapamil injection to relieve spasm.
- Try to advance the burr at 200,000 RPM into the distal lumen and withdraw the burr while spinning.
- Second arterial puncture for a second guide catheter or upsize the guide over the rota system by disassembling the Rotablator system (cut off sheath, driveshaft, and Rotawire distal to the advancer) and then try to advance a hydrophilic wire distal to the trapped burr and perform balloon dilatation of the calcified lesion proximal to the trapped burr to facilitate burr withdrawal.
- Deep intubation, either with the guide catheter or using the "mother and child" concept with subsequent pullback of all devices, can be useful to focus the force on the burr and to protect the rest of the coronary artery. By simultaneous traction on the burr shaft and countertraction on the child catheter, the catheter tip can act as a wedge between the burr and the surrounding plaque, which may exert a large and direct pulling force to retrieve the burr.
- If the above technique fails, the patient needs to be referred to CT surgery for surgical removal of the entrapped burr.

Orbital Atherectomy

Diamondback 360VR OAS by Cardiovascular Systems Inc. (CSI, St. Paul, MN) combines the principles of centrifugal force and differential sanding in the plaque modification of calcified lesions. It is an eccentrically mounted, diamond-coated 1.25 mm crown, the position of which is controlled by a control handle that orbits over a 0.012″ Viperwire™ at high speeds (Fig. 22.3). OA has the advantage of using a single device for all lesions as variation in effective burr size is based on rotational speed. It is also touted to cause less no-flow or slow-reflow phenomenon as it creates smaller particles (<2 μm in size) which are removed by the reticuloendothelial system. It reduces the risk of thermal injury to the target vessel as the elliptical orbit allows blood and microdebris to flow past and cool the crown by continuously dispersing the particulate [8].

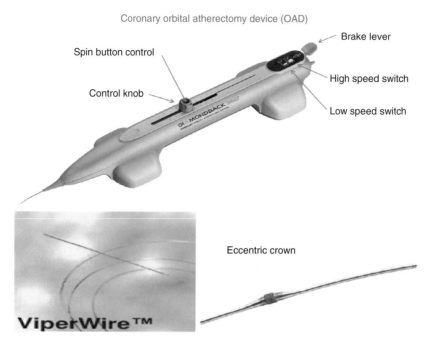

Fig. 22.3 Orbital atherectomy equipment (© Cardiovascular Systems Inc. All rights reserved. Used with the permission of Cardiovascular Systems Inc.)

Console Preparation

- Connect the spike end of saline tubing to the saline bag containing 1 litre of NS with 20 ml of ViperSlide™ lubricant (Fig. 22.4a) and connect the other end of the saline tubing luer to the OAD luer (Fig. 22.4b). Hang flush bag on to the saline pressure sensor. Make sure the pressure sensor is plugged to the back of the console. Continuous infusion of the flush solution is critical for safe coronary OA operation.
- Open the door located on the front of the OA pump and place the saline tubing in between the saline tubing positioners (Fig. 22.4c) making sure that there are no kinks and lock the door (Fig. 22.4d).
- Switch on the Master Power switch located at the back of the OA pump (Fig. 22.4e). Press the green "Start" button (Fig. 22.4f) and hold the blue "Prime" button (Fig. 22.4g) till purge solution exits the sheath near the crown (Fig. 22.4h). Ensure that there are no air bubbles in the tubing.

Initial Procedure Steps

- Cross the lesion either directly with a Viper wire or using a Fine cross miro catheter/Fielder wire exchange or using a 1.5 mm/8 OTW balloon support.
- Unlock the control knob and ensure that the crown moves freely in accordance with the movement of the control knob (Fig. 22.5a, b).

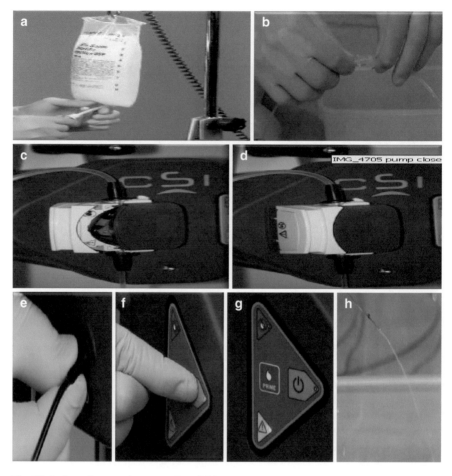

Fig. 22.4 Steps for console preparation of OA

- Move the crown control knob to 1 cm proximal (away from the shaft) (Fig. 22.5c) and release the guidewire brake (push up) (Fig. 22.5d). Thread the back end of the ViperWire through the crown, under fluoroscopic guidance (Fig. 22.5e) ensuring that the ViperWire position does not move. Position the crown approximately 1 cm proximal to the lesion.
- ViperWire spring tip should be distal to the lesion and at least 5 mm away from the rotating crown and drive shaft tip. Push down on the brake (Fig. 22.5f). The crown will not spin if the guide wire brake is not locked.
- Press and release the on/off button on top of the crown advancer knob to activate crown rotation (Fig. 22.5g). The OA is preset to low speed for all initial treatment at 80,000 RPM (Fig. 22.5h). Use low speed until device moves freely through the lesion. Then consider run(s) at high speed (120,000 RPM) (Fig. 22.5i).
- Slowly advance the crown advancer knob to begin atherectomy of the lesion at a maximum travel rate of 1 mm per second. Using fluoroscopy, verify that the crown and the crown advancer knob are moving 1:1 with one another. Slide the

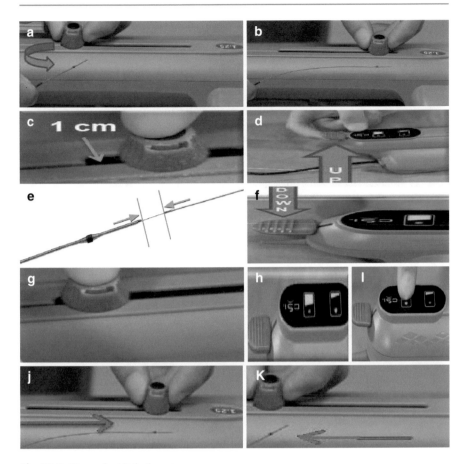

Fig. 22.5 Steps of orbital atherectomy

crown advancer knob to move the crown forward (Fig. 22.5j) and backward (Fig. 22.5k) across the lesion always returning to the proximal side of the lesion when the set is complete.

- Ensure that the OA system remains horizontal to minimize saline leakage from the OA handle. Once OA has reached full speed (as indicated by a stable pitch), do not allow the rotating crown to remain in one location as it may lead to vessel damage.
- For every 20 s of treatment, a rest period of equal time is recommended. The OA pump will emit a beep after every 25 s interval of treatment time. Maximum total treatment time should not exceed 5 min.
- After treatment, device can be removed by unlocking brake and removing over the wire ensuring that the Viperwire position remains stable under fluoroscopic guidance.

Table 22.1 for RA and OA comparison and Table 22.2 for device selection algorithm.

Table 22.1 Comparison of RA and OA

	RA	OA
Setup	Longer setup	Easier setup
Learning curve	Steeper	Shorter
Sizes	Burr can be upsized/downsized to a different size outside the body	One crown treats different vessel diameters by changing orbiting speed
Guide catheter	6 F – If burr size <1.75 mm 7 F Catheter – 2.0 burr 8 F – 2.25–2.5 burr	6 F
Use in aorto-ostial lesion	Yes	No
Use in CTO, subtotal lesions	Yes	No
Use in ISR	Yes	No
Use in distal lesions	Yes	Yes
Use in angulated lesions >90	Yes	No
Use in vessels ≥3.5 mm	Yes	No

Table 22.2 Device selection for calcific lesions

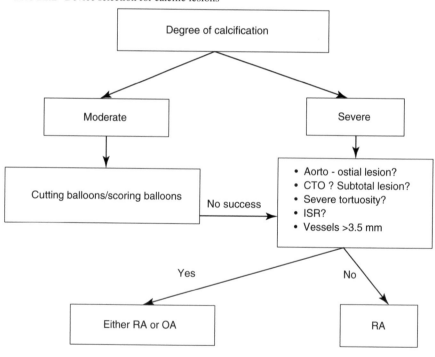

Excimer Laser Coronary Angioplasty

Laser is used in moderately calcified lesions. The X-80 laser catheter in its current form is 6 Fr (0.9 to 1.4 mm), 7Fr (1.7 mm), and 8Fr (2.0 mm) compatible and incorporates 65 concentric 50 mm fibers capable of delivering excimer energy at pulse repetition rates from 25 to 80 Hz, using a 5 s on and 10 s off cycle. This higher energy catheter maximizes tissue penetration and keeps photomechanical and photothermal damages within acceptable limits. It is expensive and not available in most cardiac catheterization labs and is inferior to RA in extremely calcified lesions [5]. Due to the predictability and high success rate with other techniques, coronary laser use has been restricted to niche applications such as debulking of undilatable and uncrossable lesions.

Cutting Balloons Atherectomy

Flextome™

The cutting balloons, which include three or four radially directed microsurgical blades on the balloon surface, create endovascular incisions in the calcium which are then further propagated with balloon inflations. Cutting balloons show greater reductions in plaque burden, yield greater luminal diameter with less inflation pressure, and cause less vascular injury compared to conventional PTCA [9–11]. The Flextome cutting balloon device consists of a nylon balloon with three (≤3 mm) or four (>3 mm) microsurgical blades mounted lengthwise on its outer surface (Fig. 22.6).

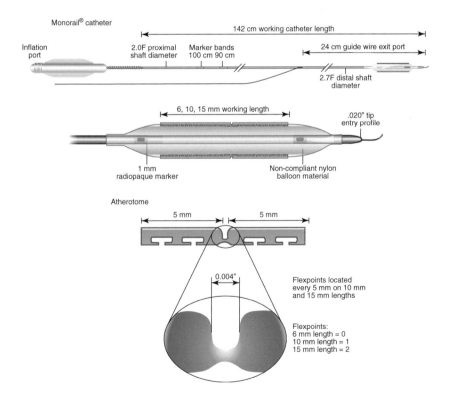

Fig. 22.6 Flextome ™ Cutting Balloon: blades mounted on a noncompliant balloon. Flex points are located every 5 mm on the balloon (© 2014 Boston Scientific Corporation or its affiliates. All rights reserved. Used with permission of Boston Scientific Corporation)

- Oversizing increases the risk of perforation. To reduce the potential for vessel damage, the inflated diameter of the Flextome Cutting Balloon Device™ should approximate a 1:1 ratio of the diameter of the vessel just proximal and distal to the stenosis.
- Maximum pressure of 8–12 atm.
- Exercise extreme care when treating a lesion distal to a stent. If the guidewire has passed through the stent cell rather than down the axis of the stent, the deflated Flextome Cutting Balloon Device could become entangled in the stent.
- When treating lesions at a bifurcation, the Flextome Cutting Balloon Device can be used prior to placing a stent, but should not be taken through the side cell of a stent to treat the side branch of a lesion at a bifurcation.

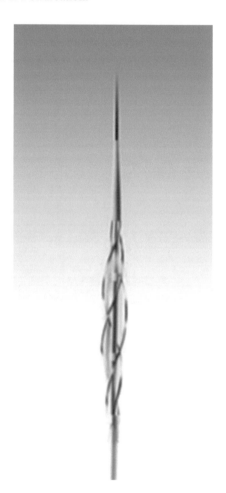

Fig. 22.7 AngioSculpt Scoring Balloon™ (© AngioScore, A Spectranetics Company. All rights Reserved. Used with the permission of Cardiovascular Systems, Inc.)

AngioSculpt™

These are flexible nitinol scoring elements with three rectangular spiral struts that work in tandem with a semi-compliant balloon to score the target lesion circumferentially with a working range of 2 atm up to 20 atm [can be tailored to vessel size]. They have a low crossing profile (~2.7 F) compatible with 6 F guiding catheters. The two radiopaque markers indicate the working ends of the balloon (Fig. 22.7).

References

1. Hoffmann R, et al. Treatment of calcified coronary lesions with Palmaz-Schatz lesions. An intravascular ultrasound study. Eur Heart J. 1998;19(8):1224–31.
2. Tan K, Sulke N, Taub N, Sowton E. Clinical and lesion morphologic determinants of coronary angioplasty success and complications: current experience. J Am Coll Cardiol. 1995;25(4):855–65.
3. Kini A, Marmur JD, Duvvuri S. Rotational atherectomy: improved procedural outcome with evolution of technique and equipment. Single-center results of first 1,000 patients. Catheter Cardiovasc Interv. 1999;46(3):305–11.
4. Dehmer GJ, Weaver D, Roe MT, Milford-Beland S, Fitzgerald S, Hermann A, Messenger J, Moussa I, Garratt K, Rumsfeld J, Brindis RG. A contemporary view of diagnostic cardiac catheterization and percutaneous coronary intervention in the United States: a report from the CathPCI Registry of the National Cardiovascular Data Registry, 2010 through June 2011. J Am Coll Cardiol. 2012;60(20):2017–31. doi:10.1016/j.jacc.2012.08.966. Epub 2012 Oct 17. PubMed PMID: 23083784.
5. Tomey MI, Kini AS, Sharma SK. Current status of rotational atherectomy. JACC Cardiov Interv. 2014;7(4):345–53.
6. Ahn SS, Auth D, Marcus DR, Moore WS. Removal of focal atheromatous lesions by angioscopically guided high-speed rotary atherectomy. Preliminary experimental observations. J Vasc Surg. 1988;7:292–300.
7. Sharma SK, Kini A, Mehran R, Lansky A, Kobayashi Y, Marmur JD. Randomized trial of rotational atherectomy versus balloon angioplasty for diffuse in-stent restenosis (ROSTER). Am Heart J. 2004;147(1):16–22.
8. Parikh K, Chandra P, Choksi N, Khanna P, Chambers J. Safety and feasibility of orbital atherectomy for the treatment of calcified coronary lesions: the ORBIT I trial. Catheter Cardiovasc Interv. 2013;81:1134–9.
9. Okura H, et al. Mechanisms of acute lumen gain following cutting balloon angioplasty in calcified and noncalcified lesions: an intravascular ultrasound study. Catheter Cardiovasc Interv. 2002;57:429–36.
10. Brown R, Kochar G, Maniet AR, Banka VS. Effects of coronary angioplasty using progressive dilation on ostial stenosis of the left anterior descending artery. Am J Cardiol. 1993;71:245–7.
11. Inoue T, et al. Lower expression of neutrophil adhesion molecule indicates less vessel wall injury and might explain lower restenosis rate after cutting balloon angioplasty. Circulation. 1998;97:2511–8.

Coronary Complications of Percutaneous Coronary Interventions

23

Mayur Lakhani, Anitha Rajamanickam, and Annapoorna Kini

This chapter discusses the common coronary complications encountered during percutaneous coronary interventions and their prevention and management.

Acute Closure

The incidence of acute closure of coronary arteries in current era is very low. Most cases of acute closure are secondary to mechanical obstruction from a dissection tissue flap and the resulting slow flow may cause activation of platelets and formation of a thrombus [1] (Fig. 23.1). Other causes of acute closure include acute thrombus formation, combination of dissection with thrombus formation, distal embolization of plaque and/or thrombus, and coronary spasm.

Angiographic risk factors for acute closure include proximal tortuosity, long lesions, heavy calcifications, degenerated vein grafts, and angulated lesions.

NHLBI Classification of Dissections [2]

- *Type A* – radiolucent areas within the coronary lumen during contrast injection, with minimal or no persistence of contrast after the dye has cleared
- *Type B* – parallel tracts or double lumen separated by a radiolucent area during contrast injection, with minimal or no persistence after dye clearance (Fig. 23.2)

M. Lakhani, MD (✉) • A. Rajamanickam, MD • A. Kini, MD, MRCP, FACC
Department of Interventional Cardiology, Mount Sinai Hospital,
One Gustave Levy Place, Madison Avenue, New York, NY 10029, USA
e-mail: drmayurlakhani@gmail.com; arajamanickam@gmail.com,
Anitha.Rajamanickam@mountsinai.org; Annapoorna.kini@mountsinai.org

© Springer-Verlag London 2014
A. Kini et al. (eds.), *Practical Manual of Interventional Cardiology*,
DOI 10.1007/978-1-4471-6581-1_23

Fig. 23.1 Pathophysiology of acute closure

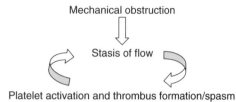

Fig. 23.2 RAO-caudal view showing type B dissection (*arrow*) in first obtuse marginal branch

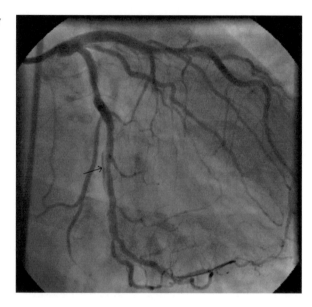

- *Type C* – contrast outside the coronary lumen, with persistence of contrast in the area after clearance of dye from the coronary lumen (Fig. 23.3)
- *Type D* – spiral luminal filling defects, frequently with extensive contrast staining of the vessel (Fig. 23.4)
- *Type E* – new, persistent filling defects
- *Type F*– dissection leading to total occlusion of the coronary artery, without distal antegrade flow

Diagnosis Acute closure is diagnosed by slow flow or absence of flow in the distal vessel commonly accompanied by chest pain, ischemic EKG changes, arrhythmias, or hypotension.

Management Acute closure should be differentiated from no-reflow. No-reflow is an acute reduction in coronary flow (TIMI grade 0–1) in a patent vessel with absence of dissection, thrombus, spasm, or high-grade residual stenosis at the original target lesion.

- Use stent delivery system (SDS) balloon or angioplasty balloon and perform Fogarty maneuver. This will dislodge any thrombus present at the site of intervention and help reestablish the flow.
- Recheck the ACT and administer additional anticoagulation to maintain ACT>300.

Fig. 23.3 RAO-caudal view showing type C dissection (*arrow*) in distal circumflex extending into first left posterolateral branch

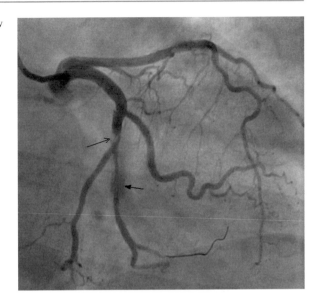

Fig. 23.4 RAO-cranial view showing type D dissection (*arrow*) with impairment of distal flow in first diagonal branch

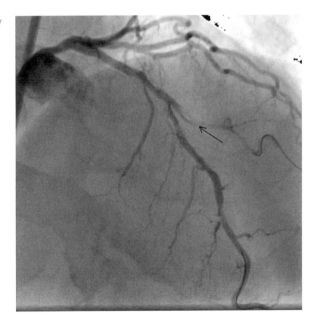

- Perform balloon angioplasty to seal the dissection flap and reestablish the flow; stabilize hemodynamics with inotropes, atropine, or IV fluid challenges. Insertion of IABP may be required. Arrhythmias should be treated with anti-arrhythmic medications and cardioversion if required.
- Perform re-stenting if dissection occurs in medium or large-sized vessels (for small-sized vessels additional balloon angioplasty may be necessary).
- If thrombus is present, use a Twin-Pass Catheter™ (Vascular Solutions) and administer distal vasodilators. Consider GP IIb-IIIa inhibitors as well.

- If above measures are ineffective, obtain multiple angiographic views to rule out air embolism, left main dissection, or distal embolization. Selective injection of contrast through the central balloon lumen or intravascular ultrasound (IVUS) may also be helpful in such cases.
- Air embolism should be managed by increasing BP using vasopressors and repeated flushing to move the air to distal microvasculature.
- Administer IV nitroglycerin if patient is hemodynamics stable (to rule out component of spasm)
- After successful reestablishment of antegrade flow, these patients require close intensive cardiac care unit monitoring.
- If none of the approaches are effective, the patient may need coronary artery bypass grafting (CABG).

Coronary No-Reflow

No-reflow is an acute reduction in coronary flow (TIMI grade 0–1) in a patent vessel with absence of dissection, thrombus, spasm, or high-grade residual stenosis at the original target lesion. The underlying mechanism is complex and not completely understood, but some proposed mechanisms include distal embolization of thrombus and/or plaque and microvascular spasm caused by release of vasoconstrictor substances like serotonin and thromboxane, oxidative stress, and reperfusion injury [3].

Clinical and lesion characteristics associated with higher incidence of no-reflow include left ventricular systolic dysfunction or hemodynamic instability, long calcified lesions, ostial lesions, chronic total occlusion of right coronary artery, thrombotic lesions, and vein graft lesions. Use of rotational atherectomy is also associated with a higher incidence of no-reflow.

Prevention Measures to prevent no-reflow include direct stenting if feasible and distal embolic protection devices for vein graft interventions. Aspiration thrombectomy in STEMI cases may help to prevent this phenomenon. For cases involving rotational atherectomy, the use of rota flush, small initial burr sizes, shorter rotablation runs, avoiding drops in rotations per minute (RPMs), and prevention of hypotension/bradycardia reduce the risk of no-reflow.

Management Differential diagnosis includes acute closure. Differentiating acute closure from no-reflow may be very challenging. Exclusion of dissection, thrombus, spasm, or high-grade residual stenosis at the original target lesion suggests no-reflow.

- Stabilize hemodynamics with medications/intra-aortic balloon pump (IABP).
- IC verapamil (100–200 μg).
- IV adenosine (10–20 μg).
- IC nitroprusside (50–200 μg).
- Moderately forceful injection of blood or saline through the manifold.
- GPIIb-IIIa agents may also be helpful.

In extreme cases of slow flow, a transit catheter or over-the-wire balloon should be used to deliver the vasodilators to the distal microvasculature. A porous balloon inflated at low pressures and delivery of GPIIb-IIIa inhibitors have shown to reduce slow flow in thrombotic lesions. In persistent cases of slow flow, insertion of IABP has shown to reduce the symptoms and subsequent periprocedural enzyme leak.

Coronary Perforation

Reported incidence of coronary perforations (CP) in 1990s and early 2000 ranged from 0.1 to 3 %. In contemporary era, the incidence is about 0.48–0.59 % [4]. Majority of contemporary cases of coronary perforations are secondary to guidewire injury, mostly from hydrophilic wires. A smaller number of cases are secondary to vessel rupture from oversized balloon/stent expansion or rotational atherectomy.

Risk Factors Angiographic characteristics associated with coronary perforations include chronic inelastic lesions (previous CABG), angulated lesions (>90), calcified lesions, and chronic total occlusions. Procedural characteristics that have been associated with an increased risk of vessel perforation include oversizing the device (balloon angioplasty or stenting) and use of an athero-ablative device (directional, rotational, orbital and excimer laser atherectomy; cutting balloon).

Classification Two classification schemes for coronary perforations are Ellis and Kini classifications. Ellis classification scheme describes wire and device perforations. Type I perforations are defined by the development of an extra luminal crater without extravasation, type II by a pericardial or myocardial blush without contrast jet extravasation, and type III by extravasation through frank ($\geq$1 mm) perforation spilling into an anatomic cavity chamber [5] (Figs. 23.5, 23.6, and 23.7). Kini scheme describes two types of wire perforations. Type I CP is described as "myocardial stain" with no frank dye extravasation and type II as "myocardial fan" with dye extravasation into pericardium, coronary sinus, or cardiac chambers [6].

Outcome Patients with Ellis/Kini type I CPs have an excellent overall prognosis. In contrast, those with Ellis type III/Kini type II CPs have a higher rate of complications and poorer long term outcomes.

Treatment Treatment depends on whether the perforation is secondary to a guidewire versus balloon/stent expansion.

- Wire perforation
  - Appropriately sized low pressure balloon inflation just proximal to the perforation site for 10 min. Confirm the vessel occlusion with contrast injection through guiding catheter.
  - Stop the anticoagulation. If bivalirudin was used for anticoagulation, stop the infusion and check the activated clotting time (ACT). If heparin was used, administer protamine sulfate for reversal (see Chapter 14).

Fig. 23.5 LAO-cranial view
showing Ellis type II/Kini
type I coronary wire
perforation

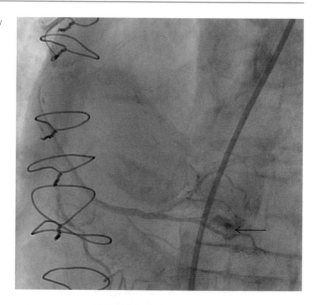

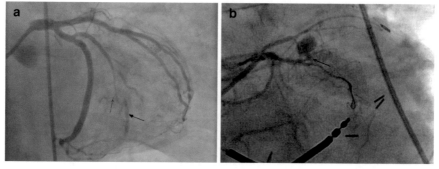

Fig. 23.6 Images showing Ellis type III/Kini type II coronary wire perforations (*arrows*)

- Deflate the balloon and obtain a cineangiogram. If continued extravasation is seen, repeat the balloon inflation for another 10 min.
- Many times up to 30 min of balloon inflation may be required to stop the extravasation. Obtain a stat transthoracic echocardiogram while the patient is still on the table to rule out a large pericardial effusion. Monitor the patient in CCU afterwards.
- In rare cases of persistent wire perforation, coil embolization of the distal vessel or exclusion of the perforated side branch by a covered (Jomed™) stent in the main vessel may be needed (see Chapter 10).
• Device perforation
  - Appropriately sized low pressure balloon inflation just proximal to the perforation site for 10 min. Confirm the vessel occlusion with contrast injection through guiding catheter.
  - Stop the anticoagulation. If bivalirudin was used for anticoagulation, stop the infusion and check the ACT. If heparin was used, administer protamine sulfate for reversal.

Fig. 23.7 RAO-caudal view showing Ellis type III coronary device perforation (*arrow*)

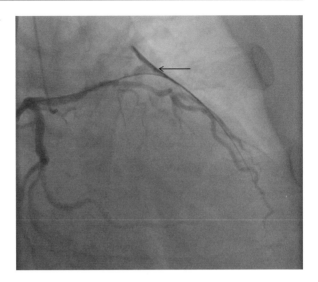

- Call for assistance. Assistant should start working on the placement of IABP and pericardiocentesis.
- If hemodynamic status is compromised, IABP should be placed by one operator while the second operator performs pericardiocentesis. Meanwhile, IV norepinephrine or vasopressin should be administered to support blood pressure.
- A covered Jomed™ stent (available in sizes from 2.8 to 4.8 mm in diameter) should be deployed to seal the perforation site as soon as possible. A 6 Fr guide will suffice for stents < 4.5 mm in diameter. For stents ≥ 4.5 mm a 7 Fr Guide is required. In cases of persistent device perforation requiring continuous balloon inflation, Jomed™ may be inserted via a second Guide catheter (from contralateral femoral access site or from the radial access site if IABP inserted already through the contralateral femoral artery) or the Guide can be upsized over the balloon delivery system if a 7 Fr Guide is required.
- Obtain a stat transthoracic echocardiogram while the patient is still on the table. Monitor the patient in CCU afterwards.

Periprocedural Myocardial Infarction (MI)

Periprocedural MI is a common complication which predicts adverse future outcomes [7].

Definition Universal definition is elevation of cardiac troponin (cTn) or CK-MB greater than five times the baseline value within 48 h of the procedure in a patient with normal baseline cTn level or rise of cTn values >20 % if the baseline values are elevated, along with evidence of prolonged ischemia as manifested by chest pain, new ischemic EKG changes, angiographic evidence of flow limiting complication/ side branch closure, or new wall motion abnormality [7]. Large periprocedural MIs are associated with an adverse long-term prognosis. Recently, Society of

Angiography and Interventions (SCAI) has proposed a new definition which recommends using elevation of isolated CK-MB $\geq 10 \times$ local laboratory upper limit of normal (ULN) or troponin $\geq 70 \times$ ULN with emphasis on CK-MB to classify periprocedural MI [8].

Common causes of periprocedural MI include acute closure, distal embolization, no-reflow, or side branch closure. It can be diagnosed by measuring cardiac biomarkers before the procedure and 3–6 h post procedure. Procedural and lesion characteristics associated with periprocedural MI include intervention on degenerated vein grafts, presence of thrombus, CTOs, long lesions, use of rotational or orbital atherectomy, prolonged balloon inflation, aggressive stent expansion, acute closure, no-reflow, and side branch closure.

Prevention The use of intravenous GPIIb-IIIa agents, p2y12 inhibitors, and statins has been shown to decrease the incidence of post-procedural MI. The use of distal embolic protection devices (EPD) for saphenous vein graft (SVG) interventions significantly reduces the periprocedural MI. For native coronary interventions, EPD have not been shown to be beneficial.

Treatment Treatment depends on the underlying cause. If there is angiographic evidence of vasospasm or slow flow, then use of IC verapamil, nitroglycerin, nitroprusside, or adenosine can be helpful. Most cases of periprocedural MI are silent. Conservative management is adequate for modest elevations in such cases. Serial enzyme measurements should be done. Patient could be discharged once the enzyme values start declining even if it remains above the baseline. For patients with persistent ischemic symptoms, EKG changes, or Q wave infarcts, repeat angiography should be considered to rule out stent thrombosis or dissection and to decide of further treatment course.

Air Embolism

Intracoronary air embolism is a potentially lethal but rare complication. It could result in hypotension, hemodynamic collapse, cardiac arrest, and in rare cases death. Coronary air embolism is almost always iatrogenic. It occurs mostly when

- Catheters are not adequately aspirated and flushed.
- During introduction or withdrawal of a guidewire, balloon catheter or other interventional devices.
- Rupture of a balloon during high inflation.
- During intracoronary medication injection.

Diagnosis Coronary air embolism is detected fluoroscopically as intracoronary filling defects during dye injection. It could also be seen as abrupt cutoff of a vessel secondary to occlusion of distal circulation with air column. Clinically small air embolism may be asymptomatic. Larger air embolism may present as chest pain, hypotension, ischemic EKG changes, or cardiac arrest.

Prevention

1. Do not engage the left main coronary when pulling out the guiding wire unless the patient has excessive aortic tortuosity or an enlarged aortic root.
2. Do not connect the manifold to the catheter with the flush running. This may lead to an air embolism if the catheter already has a column of air inside it.
3. Draw back at least 2 cc of blood into the injection syringe and make sure that the interface is free of air prior to injection.
4. Inject some dye into the ascending aorta prior to engaging left main.
5. Always ensure that all the catheters and tubings are aspirated, flushed and free of air.
6. Taking adequate care when prepping stents or balloons and ensure that the syringe tip is facing downwards.
7. Always inject with the syringe tip facing downwards.

Treatment

1. Put patient on 100 % oxygen.
2. Flush air free saline vigorously into the coronary arteries. Aspirate blood via Guide catheter and reinject forcefully back into coronary arteries.
3. Administer IV phenylephrine 200 μg for hypotension. Repeat as needed every minute. If significant hypotension or hemodynamic collapse is present, push IV 1 cc epinephrine (1:10,000 dilution).
4. Intracoronary injection of vasodilators (adenosine, nitroprusside, verapamil) may be attempted.
5. Guide wire to disrupt the air bubbles or aspiration of air bubbles using thrombectomy aspiration catheters may be attempted.
6. Supportive measures should be instituted and patient admitted to intensive coronary care unit for further monitoring.

References

1. Klein L. Coronary complications of percutaneous coronary intervention: a practical approach to the management of abrupt closure. Catheter Cardiovasc Interv. 2005;64:395–401.
2. Huber M, Mooney JF, Madison J, Mooney M. Use of a morphologic classification to predict clinical outcome after dissection from coronary angioplasty. Am J Cardiol. 1991; 68(5):467–71.
3. Piana RN, Paik GY, Moscucci M, Cohen DJ, et al. Incidence and treatment of 'no-reflow' after percutaneous coronary intervention. Circulation. 1994;89:2514–8.
4. Kiernan TJ, Yan BP, Ruggiero N, Eisenberg JD, et al. Coronary artery perforations in the contemporary interventional era. J Interv Cardiol. 2009;22:350–3.
5. Ellis SG, Ajluni S, Arnold AZ, et al. Increased coronary perforation in the new device era: incidence, classification, management, and outcome. Circulation. 1994;90:2725–30.
6. Kini AS, Rafael OC, Sarkar K, et al. Changing outcomes and treatment strategies for wire induced coronary perforations in the era of bivalirudin use. Catheter Cardiovasc Interv. 2009;74:700–7.
7. Thygesen K, Alpert JS, Jaffe AS, et al. Third universal definition of myocardial infarction. Circulation. 2012;126(16):2020.
8. Moussa ID, Klein LW, Shah B, et al. Consideration of a new definition of clinically relevant myocardial infarction after coronary revascularization. J Am Coll Cardiol. 2013;62:1563–70.

Radial Coronary Interventions

24

Christopher J. Varughese, Anitha Rajamanickam, and Robert Pyo

The radial artery access is gaining popularity due to decreased rates of access site complications and improved patient comfort. This chapter is an overview on radial interventions.

Basic Catheter Techniques for Diagnostic Angiography

Navigation

- The standard 0.035′ (150–180 cm) J wire is most commonly utilized to introduce catheters. The 0.035′ J wire has the advantage of avoiding most side branches in the forearm and arm and providing better support. The use of fluoroscopy can aid in the proper passage of these wires into the ascending aorta without engaging side branches (carotids, vertebrals, mammary, etc.).
- The 0.035′ Angled Glide Terumo Wire (Terumo®, Tokyo, Japan) can be used to navigate tortuous vasculature.

C.J. Varughese, MD (✉) • A. Rajamanickam, MD • R. Pyo, MD
Department of Interventional Cardiology, Mount Sinai Hospital,
One Gustave Levy Place, Madison Avenue, New York, NY 10029, USA
e-mail: cvarughese@gmail.com; arajamanickam@gmail.com,
Anitha.Rajamanickam@mountsinai.org; Robert.pyo@mountsinai.org

© Springer-Verlag London 2014
A. Kini et al. (eds.), *Practical Manual of Interventional Cardiology*,
DOI 10.1007/978-1-4471-6581-1_24

Pearl

The 0.035 J wire is the safest wire to use and will be effective in over 90 % of cases. If a glide wire is needed, be sure to use a curved-tip wire and utilize fluoroscopy to guide progress of the wire. In difficult cases a 0.014′ Grandslam wire may be used.

If the wire or catheter does not progress easily, be aware of several possibilities:[1]

Spasm

Small radial artery

Loops

High takeoff

Remnant artery

Stenosis

Side branch

Radial Diagnostic Catheters

- Judkins Left (JL)[2] or Judkins Right (JR)
- Specialized radial catheters – Tiger and Jacky (Terumo®, Tokyo, Japan)

Cannulation Note that described maneuvers to engage catheters in this section are performed in the left anterior oblique (LAO) 20–30°.

- Left Main (LM) Coronary Artery
    - After obtaining access, gently advance a J wire (standard length or exchange length J wire), and with the aid of fluoroscopy, traverse the aortic arch and advance to the level of the aortic arch.
    - Advance the JL 3.5 catheter to the level of the transverse aortic arch; ask the patient to take a deep breath and advance the J wire to the level of the aortic valve. If the J wire does not automatically advance into the left coronary sinus, use the JL catheter to direct the J wire into the proper sinus. Advance the JL catheter into the left coronary sinus and withdraw the J wire.
    - Gentle clock or counter clock rotations combined with a gentle forward push will result in successful cannulation.
    - After completion of LCA angiography, the JL 3.5 catheter is disengaged from the left main coronary artery, and an exchange length 0.035′ J wire is advanced to the level of the aortic valve and the JL catheter is extracted over the wire.

[1] See "Troubleshooting."

[2] Note: When utilizing the Judkins catheters, successful cannulation of the left main coronary artery will more easily be achieved with a Judkins catheter that is 0.5 size smaller than that chosen for the transfemoral approach.

- Right Coronary Artery (RCA)
  - Advance the JR4 catheter over the exchange wire to the right or left coronary sinus and remove the J wire.
  - If catheter is in the left coronary sinus, pull and turn the catheter clockwise to place it in the right coronary sinus.
  - A clockwise rotation of the JR4 catheter will enable proper cannulation.
- LIMA and RIMA
  - Obtaining access on the ipsilateral side of the bypass graft will be the easiest approach.
  - Advance J wire across the subclavian.
  - Advance JR4 catheter (or internal mammary) catheter beyond LIMA graft or RIMA graft.
  - Pull back wire into catheter and pull back catheter and engage graft.
- Left Ventricular (LV) Angiography
  - Left ventriculography is performed in the same approach as that of the femoral artery.
  - No special sizing adjustment for the pigtail catheter is necessary.

Specialized Catheters

- Catheters made specifically for radial procedures include the Tiger and Jacky.
- Advantage: They can be used to engage both the left main and right coronary arteries and thus obviate need for exchange to a second catheter.
- Disadvantage: Require specific experience in maneuvering to use them effectively and safely.

Pearls
When using the right radial approach, left-sided catheters have to be downsized. Catheters to engage the right coronary artery often have to be longer (i.e., Amplatz right catheters instead of Judkins right catheters may have to be used). No size adjustment is necessary when using the left radial approach.

   If there is trouble engaging a coronary artery, be aware that it is difficult to "make" a catheter work during a radial approach. It is often easier to try another catheter.

Transradial PCI

Guiding Catheter Selection

- When using a right radial access, choose a left guiding catheter that is 0.5 smaller than a guide that would be chosen if a femoral artery access is utilized (i.e., if a Mach 1 VL 3.5 guide would have been used for a femoral approach, the radial equivalent

is a Mach 1 VL 3.0). A longer right coronary guide may be required. Amplatz guides may be useful when performing right coronary artery interventions.
- No size adjustment is necessary if a left radial access is used.
- Specialized guides for radial interventions include the Ikari guides (Terumo®, Tokyo, Japan). These specialized guides are designed for optimal support during radial interventions.

Other Equipment

- The same guidewires, balloons, and stents that are typically used for the femoral artery are also utilized for transradial interventions.
- Specialized interventional devices including rotational atherectomy devices can also be used safely during transradial interventions.

Pearl
Size adjustments in guide selection are required when using the right radial artery. No guide size adjustment is necessary when using the left radial artery.

Post Procedure Care

- Hemostasis – The Terumo® TR Band™ is a device designed to achieve hemostasis for the transradial approach.
  - Choose appropriate TR Band size (regular or large).
  - Wrap TR Band around wrist and secure in place via Velcro band.
  - A small green box indicates where the band should be placed proximal to the radial percutaneous site.
  - Instill 15 cc of air. Then remove air 1 cc at a time until bleeding occurs at which time 1–2 cc of air is reinjected into the balloon. The idea is to achieve hemostasis without completing occluding the radial artery.
  - Save the syringe for future deflation.
- TR Band Removal
  - Air removal can begin 120 min after the sheath is pulled (4 h for PCI).
  - Once it is time to remove the TR Band, the operator should withdraw 1 cc of air at a time that was initially instilled into the balloon and observe for any bleeding.
  - If bleeding occurs, reinject air that was removed until hemostasis is achieved, and reattempt deflation in 30 min.
  - If no bleeding is observed, the operator should remove all air and deflate the balloon completely and observe for bleeding. If there is no bleeding, the operator can remove the TR Band and place a protective covering (i.e., Tegaderm™) over the radial percutaneous site.
  - Vital signs and pulse check q 15 min×4, q 30 min×2, and q 1 h until post sheath removal. Assess for presence of feeling in the fingers and capillary refill in distal fingers and nail beds until TR Band is removed.

> **Pearl**
> When placing a hemostatic device after a radial intervention, avoid occlusion of the radial artery. Applying just enough pressure to achieve hemostasis is essential to avoid post procedure radial artery occlusion.

Discharge Instructions

- Limit bending of affected wrist for 24 h.
- No lifting of greater than 5 lbs with affected hand for 5 days.
- No bathing showering or driving for 24 h.

Troubleshooting

Spasm

- Minimize pain and administer additional sedatives.
- Repeat administration of intra-arterial nitroglycerin (200 mcg) and/or verapamil (250 mcg).
- Apply a warm compress over the forearm.
- If sheath removal is not possible due to radial artery spasm around it, wait 1 h and administer additional sedatives/analgesics and reattempt.
- Persistent radial artery spasm preventing sheath removal may require deep sedation with the assistance of an anesthesiologist.

Subclavian Loop

- Navigate the loop with 0.035′ wire glide wire.
- Advance diagnostic or guide catheter over the wire.
- Once the catheter has passed beyond the loop, a counterclockwise rotation while pulling back will straighten the loop.
- For extreme tortuosity, it may be necessary to cannulate the LCA/RCA with the 0.035′ wire within the catheter.
- Only attempt to manipulate the catheter for cannulation with loop straightened. If the loop was reformed, repeat step 3. It will be extremely difficult to manipulate the catheter with a loop present.

Radial Artery Tortuosity and Loops

- Perform selective angiography to identify the problem.
- Utilize hydrophilic 0.035 Terumo glide wire or 0.014 coronary guidewire to navigate the loop or tortuosity.
- Advance a hydrophilic catheter over the wire and then apply a gentle counterclock rotation while pulling back the catheter to straighten the loop.
- Exchange out the first wire with a work J wire.

Arteria Lusoria (Lusorian Artery) The innominate artery arises from the descending portion of the thoracic aorta.

- It is difficult to pass a catheter into the ascending aorta. Other problems include difficult cannulation of the coronary arteries.
- Advance the catheter into the ascending aorta (LAO 60).
- Ask the patient for a deep inspiration and attempt to advance wire into ascending aorta.
- If the wire only goes down the descending aorta, push the catheter into the descending aorta, pull wire and slowly withdraw catheter, and direct it into the ascending aorta with rotation.
- Be prepared to choose an alternate site of vascular access. This anatomy is associated with one of the highest rates for transradial intervention failure.

Catheter Kinking

- Rotate under fluoroscopy in a direction opposite of what caused the kink.
- Gentle forward or backward movement of the catheter will facilitate unkinking rotation.
- Whenever possible, pass a 0.035″ Terumo® guidewire beyond the kinked portion to facilitate removal of the catheter in one piece.

Complications [1–4]

Radial Artery Occlusion

- Prevention: Transradial cocktail
- Prevention: Nonocclusive bandage (dedicated radial compression set)
- Treatment: Angioplasty in symptomatic cases

Radial Artery Pseudoaneurysm

- Treatment: US guided compression bandage
- Treatment: US guided thrombin injection

Brachial Artery (BA) or Subclavian Artery (SA) Dissection

- Prevention: Never advance the catheter without GW.
- Prevention: Be cautious in excessive brachial or subclavian tortuosity.
- Treatment: Prolonged balloon dilation and stenting of flow limiting dissections.

Reflex Sympathetic Dystrophy

- Very rare – likely a result of prolonged and aggressive compression
- Treatment: Multimodality approach utilizing medical pain management and physical therapy

Hematoma, Perforation, and Compartment Syndrome

- Predisposing Factors
  - Anticoagulated state
  - Small vessels
  - Low BMI
  - Women
  - Diabetic
  - Older patients
  - Spasm
  - Tortuosity and remnants of radial artery
  - Use of hydrophilic guidewires
- Avoidance
  - Avoid use of force when wiring.
  - Utilize fluoroscopic or angiographic guidance (especially when using glide wires).
  - Avoid forceful injections as it may cause hydraulic perforation.
  - Attempt to straighten tortuosity with 0.014 guidewire first.
  - Use a J wire whenever possible.
- Perforation Management: During Procedure
  - Upsize the radial sheath for a longer, larger diameter one that will cover the perforated portion of the vessel. This maneuver may tamponade and actually seal the perforation. However, be aware of severe spasm.
  - Position BP cuff after catheter passage and inflate BP cuff 20 mmHg below SBP. Monitor finger O_2 saturation during inflated BP cuff. Deflate BP cuff every 15 min.
- Perforation Management: Post Procedure
  - In addition to above, consider second compression device (i.e., elastic band).
  - Reverse anticoagulation.
  - Manual compression.
  - Consult vascular surgery for large perforations to help manage potential compartment syndrome and circulatory compromise.

Hematoma Classification After Transradial/Ulnar PCI

- Grade I – Local hematoma, superficial
- Grade II – Hematoma with moderate muscular infiltration
- Grade III – Forearm hematoma and muscular infiltration below the elbow
- Grade IV – Hematoma and muscular infiltration extending beyond the elbow
- Grade V – Ischemic threat (compartment syndrome)

Conclusions

The cornerstone to a successful radial artery percutaneous intervention involves a systematic and stepwise approach. Increasing operator experience and knowledge of pitfalls will lead to easier cannulation and shorter procedure times.

References

1. Hammon M, Pristipino C, Di Mario C, et al. Consensus document on the radial approach in percutaneous cardiovascular intervention: Position paper by the European Association of Percutaneous Cardiovascular Interventions and the Working groups on Acute Cardiac Care and Thrombosis of the European Society of Cardiology. EuroIntervention. 2013;8:1242–51.
2. Caputo RP, Tremmel JA, Rao S, et al. Transradial arterial access for coronary and peripheral procedures: Executive summary by the Transradial Committee of the SCAI. Catheter Cardiovasc Interv. 2011;78:823–39.
3. Wilkins RG. Radial artery cannulation and ischemic damage. A review. Anaesthesia. 1985;40:896–9.
4. Rao SV, Tremmel JA, Gilchrist IC, et al. Best practices for transradial angiography and intervention: a consensus statement from the Society for Cardiovascular Angiography and Intervention's Transradial Working group. Catheter Cardiovasc Interv. 2014;83(2):228–36.

Part III

Special Procedures

Advanced Hemodynamic Support

25

Anitha Rajamanickam and Annapoorna Kini

The dramatic advances in the field of interventional cardiology have resulted in the shift toward PCI as opposed to CABG in high-risk complex lesions, especially surgically nonamenable lesions. Use of LV assist devices have increased the odds of success and decreased mortality, morbidity, and overall health-care costs [1–3]. Cardiogenic shock complicates 7–10 % of STEMI and the key cause of in-hospital mortality [4]. Unloading of the myocardium mechanically may limit infarct size, maintain end organ perfusion and decrease myocardial oxygen demand [5–7].

Available Commonly Used Advanced Hemodynamic Support

A good percutaneous circulatory support device should be easily placed without significant complications and provide output of >2 L/mt for hours to days without an external blood circuit. See Table 25.1 for indications of hemodynamic support in PCI. The two commonly used are IABP and Impella 2.5 LP system/CP system (Abiomed). TandemHeart is now infrequently used. Table 25.2 shows our selection algorithm for the type of hemodynamic support device.

A. Rajamanickam, MD (✉) • A. Kini, MD, MRCP, FACC
Department of Interventional Cardiology, Mount Sinai Hospital,
One Gustave Levy Place, Madison Avenue, New York, NY 10029, USA
e-mail: arajamanickam@gmail.com, Anitha.Rajamanickam@mountsinai.org;
Annapoorna.kini@mountsinai.org

© Springer-Verlag London 2014

233

A. Kini et al. (eds.), *Practical Manual of Interventional Cardiology*,
DOI 10.1007/978-1-4471-6581-1_25

Table 25.1 Indications for hemodynamic support in PCI

Indications
Cardiogenic shock
Severely compromised LV dysfunction
Mechanical complications of an AMI
Complex coronary lesions (such as unprotected left main disease, complex multivessel disease, last remaining conduit vessel, and bypass graft disease)
As a bridge to further therapy
Prophylaxis in patients with severe left main coronary arterial stenosis
Intractable myocardial ischemia
Refractory heart failure
Intractable ventricular arrhythmias

Table 25.2 Algorithm for LV support device use

LVEF	Simple PCI	Complex PCI
>35 %	No support	IABP
20–35 %	IABP	Impella/TandemHeart
<20 %	Impella/TandemHeart	Impella/TandemHeart

The Intra-aortic Balloon Pump (IABP) (Fig. 25.1)

IABP is used in 30 % of patients undergoing complex PCIs in the United States. It is an over-the-wire balloon catheter that has a fiberoptic sensor for beat to beat adjustment and accuracy. It requires a certain residual level of left ventricular function to be effective. It continues to be a favorite owing to quick and easy implantation, relatively low cost, and a low complication rate. Potential complications are listed in Table 25.3.

Contraindications

- Severe aortic insufficiency
- Aortic aneurysm
- Aortic dissection
- Limb ischemia

Balloon Size

- 35 cm balloon if patient's height is <5 ft
- 40 cm balloon if patient's height is between 5 and 6 ft (*most commonly used*)
- 50 cm balloon if patient's height is >6 ft

Access

- Obtain optimal femoral access or use preexisting access to place the 7 Fr or 8 Fr sheath that comes with balloon pump kit (see Chap. 1).

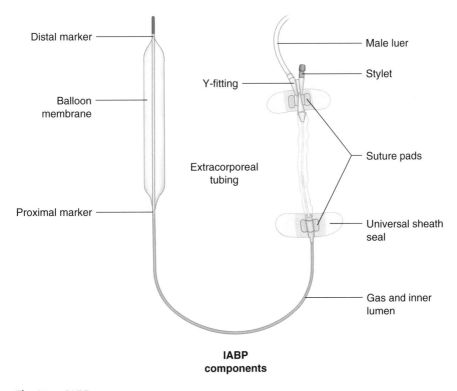

Fig. 25.1   IABP

Table 25.3   Potential complications of IABP

Potential complications			
Access site complications	Aortic dissection	Limb ischemia	Thrombocytopenia
Refer to Chap. 1			
Bleeding			Check CBC daily
Infection	Prevent by inserting balloon over wire	Avoid by using the smallest sheath size and use the limb with the strongest pulse	Asses for HIT
Vascular complications	Assess daily for pain between shoulder blades	Use Xylocaine for spasm	Decrease or stop heparin
Compartment syndrome	Remove IABP and surgery for repair if needed	Bypass graft for the affected extremity if needed and change insertion site to opposite limb	Transfuse platelets as needed

- Sheathless in morbid obesity or scarring of the groin.
- Use a shallow angle of insertion <45.°
- Advance catheter in small steps of less than 1 in. at a time to avoid kinking.
- If kinking is suspected, reposition by pulling back ½ in.

Balloon Preinsertion Preparation

- Open the tray and do not remove balloon from T handle sheath.
- Attach the one-way valve to male Luer fitting of IABP catheter (Fig. 25.2) and a 60 cc syringe.
- Negative pressure on balloon (about 30 cc) ×2 with the balloon tip remaining inside the sheath and detach the syringe only leaving the one-way valve in place of the IABP (Fig. 25.3).

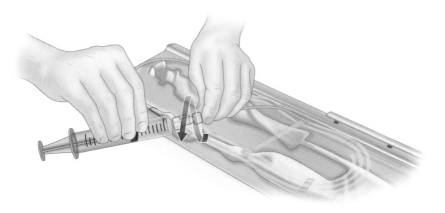

Fig. 25.2 Attach the one-way valve to main Luer fitting of IABP catheter and a 60 cc syringe

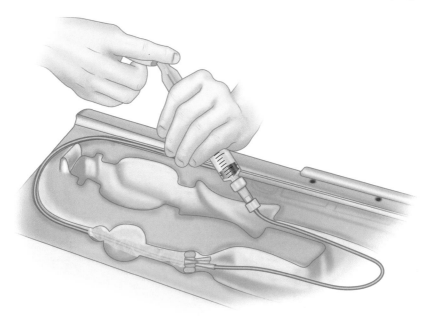

Fig. 25.3 Negative pressure on balloon

- Remove stylet, and flush the inner lumen with 3–5 cc of flush solution. Elevate flush bag at least 3 ft above transducer and connect to pressure @ 300 mmHg to maintain a 3 cc/h continuous flow through inner lumen of the IABP (Fig. 25.4).

Balloon Insertion

- Place a 8Fr catheter in femoral artery (see Chap. 1) with needle insertion at <45° angle (Fig. 25.5).
- Remove IABP by pulling straight from the T handle. Do not dip, wipe, or handle membrane prior to insertion (Fig. 25.6).

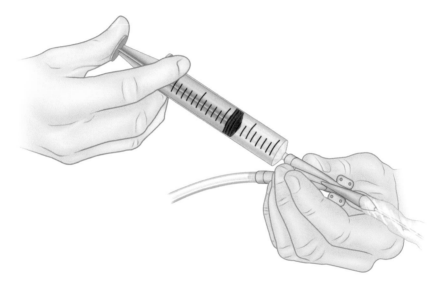

Fig. 25.4 Flush the inner lumen

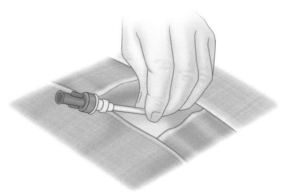

Fig. 25.5 Insert 8 Fr sheath

- Advance 0.018″ wire to level of aortic arch. Using small short movements, advance the balloon over the wire till the distal tip is at the level of carina. Proximal tip should be above renal arteries.
- Advance sheath seal as far as possible into the hub of sheath and secure IABP catheter to patient's leg using STATLOCK® or sutures (Fig. 25.7).
- Remove guidewire, aspirate back 3–5 cc of blood from inner lumen and flush with another 5 cc of flush solution (Fig. 25.8).

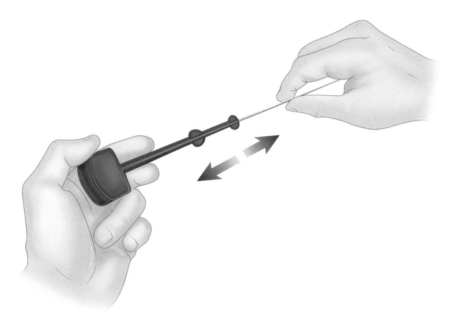

Fig. 25.6 Remove IABP by pulling straight

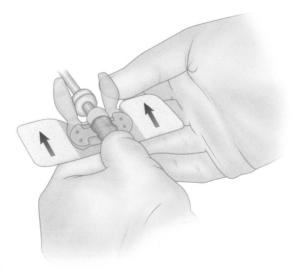

Fig. 25.7 Secure IABP with STATLOCK® or sutures

- Remove one-way valve from IABP catheter and attach male Luer to female Luer fitting of Pneumatic Module of IABP. Hand over fiberoptic cable, if IABP is fiberoptic, to the technician (Fig. 25.10)

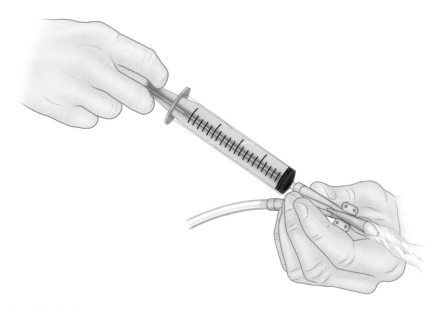

Fig. 25.8 Flush catheter

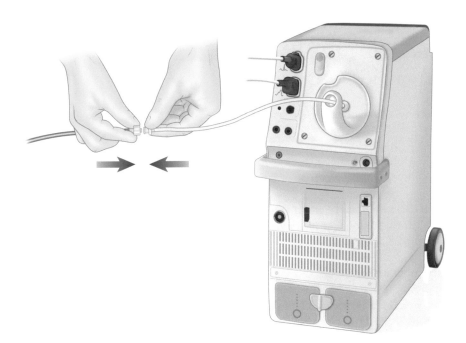

Fig. 25.9 Attach male Luer to female Luer fitting of Pneumatic Module of IABP

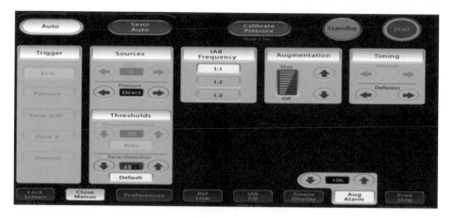

Fig. 25.10 Press "start button," select mode, and set frequency at 1:1

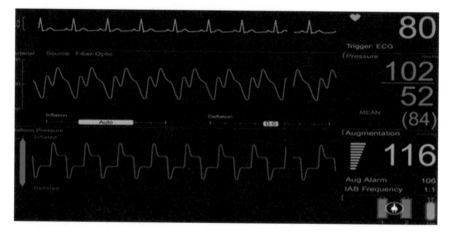

Fig. 25.11 IAB frequency confirmed on console

- Press "start button"
  - Select mode:
    - *Auto Mode*: Automatically selects most appropriate lead and trigger and sets the inflation and deflation timing
    - *Asynchronous*: Rate of 80/mt and only used when patient has no cardiac output
  - Select frequency: at 1:1 (Fig. 25.10)
- Confirm fluoroscopic balloon inflation and the balloon waveforms on the console (Fig. 25.11)

Troubleshooting Inflation occurs at the dicrotic notch as a sharp "V" and ideally diastolic augmentation rises above systole (Fig. 25.12). Deflation occurs just prior to systolic ejection and results in a reduction in assisted end-diastolic and end-systolic pressure (Fig. 25.12). See Fig. 25.13 for variations with heart rate and rhythm.

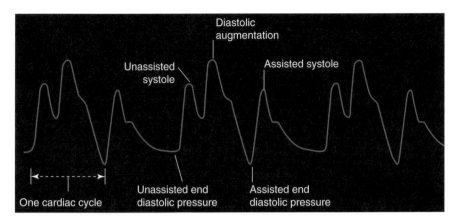

Fig. 25.12 Inflation of the IABP occurs at the dicrotic notch and deflation occurs just prior to systolic ejection

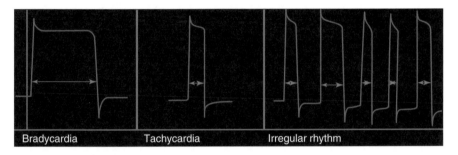

Fig. 25.13 Normal variations in balloon pressure waveform

Timing Errors: Adjust Onset of Inflation/Deflation

- *Early inflation prior to aortic valve closure or dicrotic notch*
  - Diastolic augmentation encroaches onto systole and causes AI and increase in LVEDP and MVO_2 demand (Fig. 25.14)
- *Early deflation during diastolic phase*
  - Deflation is seen as a sharp drop following diastolic augmentation (Fig. 25.15) and causes suboptimal coronary perfusion, retrograde coronary and carotid blood flow, and increased MVO_2 demand.
- *Late inflation markedly after dicrotic notch*
  - This causes suboptimal diastolic augmentation and coronary artery perfusion (Fig. 25.16).
- *Late deflation after aortic valve has opened*
  - Afterload reduction is essentially absent (Fig. 25.17) and MVO_2 consumption is increased and may impede left ventricular ejection.

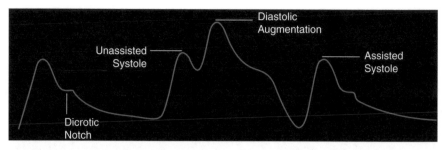

Fig. 25.14 Early IABP inflation prior to aortic valve closure or the dicrotic notch

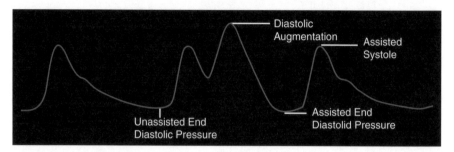

Fig. 25.15 Early IABP deflation during diastolic phase

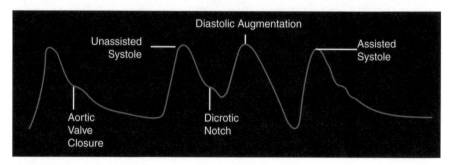

Fig. 25.16 Late inflation markedly after dicrotic notch

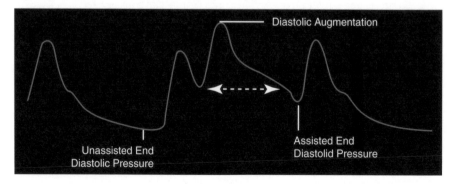

Fig. 25.17 Late deflation after aortic valve has opened

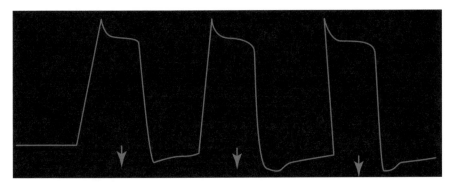

Fig. 25.18 Gas loss

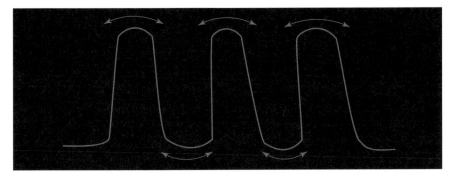

Fig. 25.19 Catheter restriction

Gas Loss (Fig. 25.18)

If blood observed
- Stop pumping and remove IABP.

If blood not observed
- Check if connections are tight, perform an autofill, and press start.

Catheter Restriction (Fig. 25.19)

Restriction in IABP or tubing
- Relieve restriction.

Membrane not unfolded
- Try to manually inflate/deflate.

IABP remains in sheath
- Make sure IABP is in position.

Impella

Catheter-based, impeller-driven, axial flow pump which pumps blood directly from the LV into the ascending aorta for up to 5 days *and* up to 2.5 L/min of CO for Impella 2.5 and 4 L/min for Impella CS

Contraindications

- Mural thrombus in the left ventricle
- Mechanical aortic valve or moderate to severe aortic stenosis (AVA of ≤ 1.5 cm^2)
- Moderate to severe aortic insufficiency (echocardiographic grade $\geq 2+$)
- Abdominal aneurysms
- Severe peripheral vascular disease or extreme tortuosity/calcifications
- Renal failure (creatinine ≥ 4 mg/dL)
- Liver dysfunction (platelet count $\leq 75,000$/mm^3 or INR ≥ 2.0 or fibrinogen ≤ 1.50 g/L)
- Recent (<3 months) stroke or TIA

Preimplantation

- Iliofemoral angiography to rule out severe PVD.
- Deploy 2 preclose sutures (see VCD Devices).
- Press power side button of console for 3 s. Console automatically performs a system check (Fig. 25.20).
- Open the Impella kit under sterile conditions (Fig. 25.21).

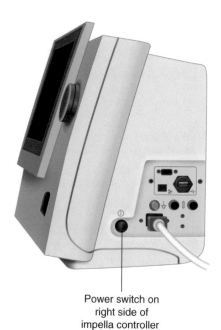

Power switch on
right side of
impella controller

Fig. 25.20 Press power button for 3 s

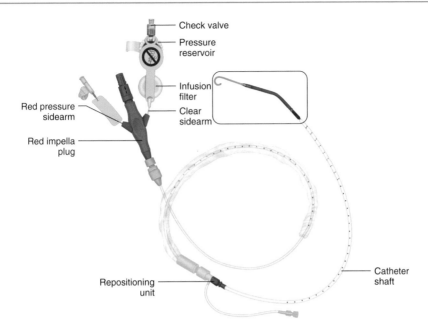

Fig. 25.21 Open Impella kit

- Press "menu" and "start case"
- *Auto prime* [performed by the nonsterile technician]
  - Connect purge fluid spike of the purge cassette to the purge fluid bag [500 ml of 20 % dextrose + heparin 50 U/ml] (Fig. 25.22).
  - Press open the purge cassette door on the left side of the console, and snap the purge cassette into the slot, then slide the purge pressure transmitter to the right till you hear a snap (Fig. 25.23).
  - Controller automatically starts to prime the purge cassette.
- *Auto detect*
  - Connect the black end of connector cable (Fig. 25.24) to the red Impella catheter (Fig. 25.24). Snap the clear plastic clip on the side arm to the connector cable (Fig. 25.26).
  - Hand the white end of the white connector cable to the technician to connect to the console with a click as shown. Controller automatically recognizes the catheter type (Fig. 25.25).
- *Auto de-air*
  - Connect the red port of the purge system to the red port of the Impella catheter and the yellow port of the system to the yellow port of the Impella catheter (Fig. 25.27). Ensure connections are tight.
  - Squeeze the white flush valve for 10 s till controller beeps and fluid exits the Impella catheter (Fig. 25.28). Screen will show "Catheter is ready to insert." Select "default" for purge fluid values.

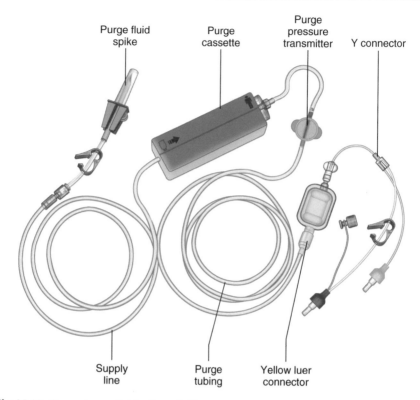

Fig. 25.22 Connect purge fluid spike to fluid

Implantation

- Insert a 7 F introducer/catheter and remove the introducer. Administer heparin to achieve an ACT of 250–300 s or bivalirudin to achieve an ACT of >300 s.
- After successive dilations with 8Fr, 10Fr, and 12Fr dilators (Fig. 25.29), upgrade to a 13Fr [Impella 2.5] or 14Fr [Impella CP] peel away catheter/dilator by supporting the shaft of the introducer (Fig. 25.30).
- Remove the 13 or 14 Fr dilator and insert a 6 Fr diagnostic catheter (Judkins Right or Multipurpose with no side holes) over a 0.035″ guidewire into the left ventricle (Fig. 25.31).
- Exchange the 0.035 wire for a 0.018 guidewire and advance it till the floppy end and 3–4 cm of the stiffer part are visible in the left ventricle. Remove the 6 Fr diagnostic catheter.
- Backload the blue pigtail section on a 0.014 guidewire using preassembled EasyGuide Red lumen until it exits near the label (Fig. 25.32).
- Remove EasyGuide by gently pulling the label while holding the Impella® catheter (Fig. 25.33).

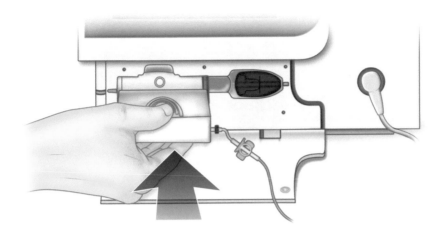

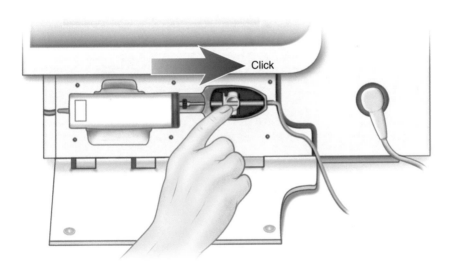

Fig. 25.23 Snap purge cassette into slot

- Keep the wire parallel to the cannula and advance the catheter in small increments to avoid bending the cannula (Fig. 25.34).
- Advance the catheter into the middle of LV, without coiling the guidewire, under fluoroscopy to 4 cm below the AV annulus free from mitral valve chordae. Ensure that the Impella is positioned across the aortic valve with the pigtail and inlet portion in the left ventricle and the outlet and motor portion in the aorta. Align catheter against the lesser curvature of aorta (Fig. 25.35).

Fig. 25.24 Connect connector cable to Impella

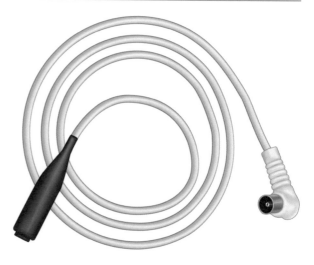

White connector cable

Fig. 25.25 Connect cable to console

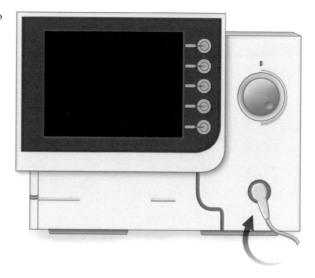

- Remove any excess slack. Confirm that an aortic waveform is displayed on the Impella Console (Fig. 25.36). At the end of the procedure, the Impella catheter can be safely removed from the LV.

Troubleshooting If the Impella® catheter advances too far into the LV and the controller displays a ventricular waveform (Fig. 25.37), pull the catheter back until an aortic waveform is present. As soon as the aortic waveform appears, pull the catheter back an additional 4 cm (the distance between adjacent markings on the catheter is 1 cm).

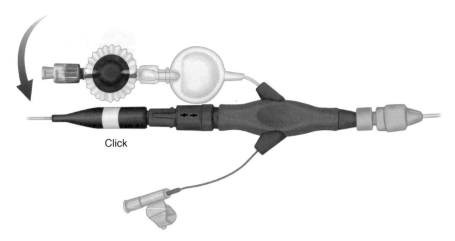

Fig. 25.26 Snap clear plastic clip on the side arm

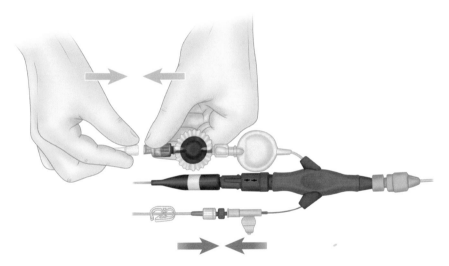

Fig. 25.27 Connect Impella to purge system

Potential Complications

- Access site complications.
- Bleeding complications.
- Displacement of the pump back into the aorta can also occur, but the addition of the pigtail catheter tip minimizes the displacement potential (see trouble shooting above).

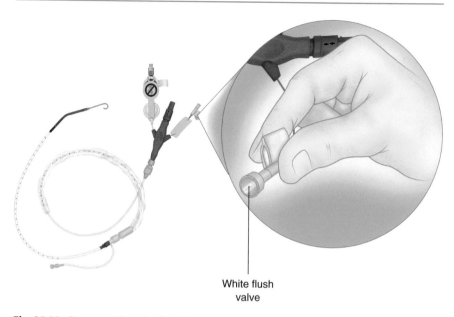

White flush
valve

Fig. 25.28 Squeeze white valve for 10 s till controller beeps and fluid exits the Impella

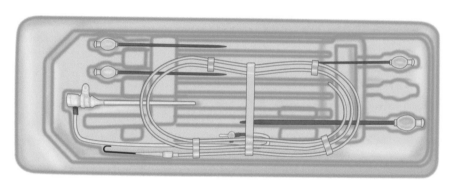

Fig. 25.29 Successively dilate to 12 Fr

- In a recent meta-analysis, hemolysis as measured by free hemoglobin was significantly higher. Also noted was a trend toward higher rates of PRBC and plasma transfusion with Impella as compared to IABP [8].

TandemHeart

The TandemHeart (TH) is a left atrial-to-femoral bypass percutaneous ventricular assist device that can provide rapid short-term left ventricular support which comprises of:

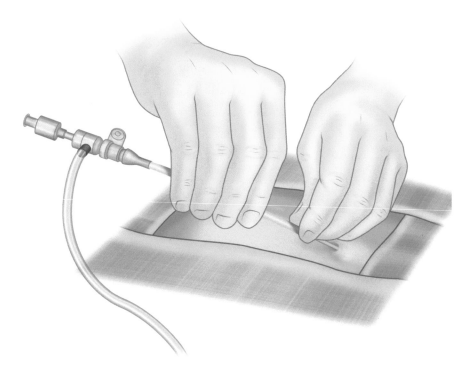

Fig. 25.30 Upgrade to a 13Fr catheter/dilator

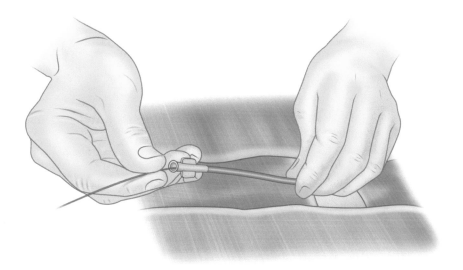

Fig. 25.31 Insert 0.035″ guidewire into LV

Fig. 25.32 EasyGuide Red
lumen

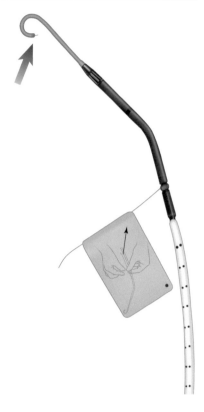

- 21 Fr venous transseptal inflow cannula to aspirate oxygenated blood from the left atrium [LA]
- Continuous flow centrifugal blood pump delivering up to 5.0 l/min
- 15–17 Fr arterial sheaths to pump blood from LA to right femoral artery or two 12 Fr arterial perfusion catheters to pump blood into the right and left femoral arteries

The Tandem heart pump comprises of a:

- Unique lubrication system, which feeds a nominal 10 cc/h of heparinized saline to cool the motor.
- Pressure transducer that monitors the infusion pressure and identifies any disruption in the infusion line.
- In-line air bubble detector that monitors for the presence of air in the infusion line.

Contraindications

- Ventricular septal defect
- Aortic insufficiency
- Severe PVD

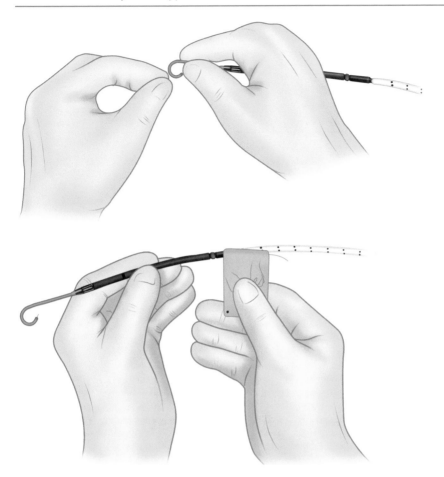

Fig. 25.33 Remove EasyGuide by gently pulling the label while holding the Impella

Steps of Implantation

- Iliofemoral angiography to rule out severe PVD.
- Femoral artery access and preclosure with the Perclose™ device (see VCD Devices) upsize to a 15–17 Fr arterial sheath.
- Transseptal puncture (see Chap. 27) via femoral vein under fluoroscopic guidance using the Brockenbrough needle and a Mullins sheath is performed and its position in the LA is confirmed.
- Unfractionated heparin to achieve an ACT >400 s
- Exchange Mullins sheath for the 21 Fr TH transseptal cannula with the 14 Fr obturator over the 0.038 in. J-tip 260 cm Amplatz Super Stiff guidewire and confirm its position [ensure all side holes of the TH are in the LA] by injecting dye and assessing the blood oxygen saturation level.

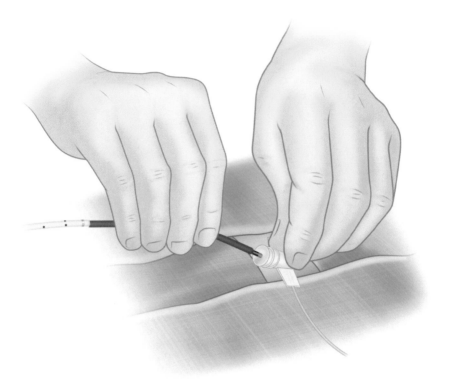

Fig. 25.34 Advance the catheter in small increments to avoid bending the cannula

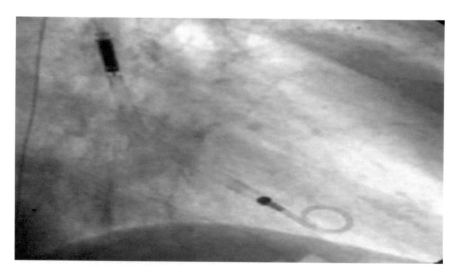

Fig. 25.35 Advance the catheter into the middle of LV

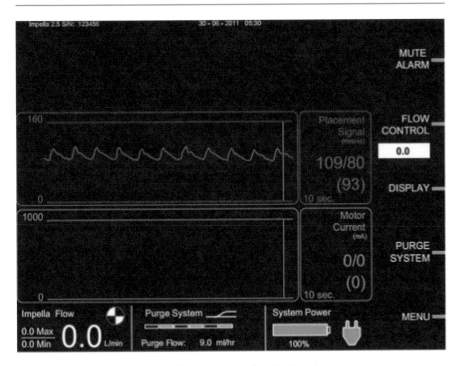

Fig. 25.36 An Aortic waveform is displayed on the Impella Console

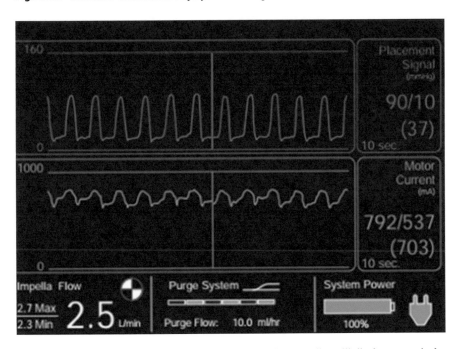

Fig. 25.37 If the Impella advances too far into the LV, the controller will display a ventricular waveform

- The obturator and the wire are then removed and clamps applied for temporary homeostasis. Suture the peripheral end of the cannula to the skin of the patient's thigh and clamp it.
- Place the 15 Fr arterial perfusion cannula of the TH device with the distal end of the cannula lying above the aortic bifurcation. Suture the peripheral end to the patient's thigh and clamp it.
- De-air the extracorporeal system and attach the TH cannula to the inflow port of the centrifugal blood pump and femoral arterial cannula to the outflow conduit of the TH pump in the standard wet-to-wet fashion with Tygon tubing. Connect power supply to the microprocessor-based controller.
- Connect the pump to the TH controller and adjust the speed to provide a cardiac output of 2.5–3.0 L/min.

Complications

- Puncture/rupture of aortic root, coronary sinus, or posterior free wall of the right atrium.
- Thromboembolism – Unfractionated heparin to maintain an activated clotting time of 400 s during insertion and 250–300 s during support is mandatory.
- Hypothermia.
- Access site complications.

References

1. Valgimigli M, et al. Sirolimus-eluting versus paclitaxel-eluting stent implantation for the percutaneous treatment of left main coronary artery disease: a combined RESEARCH and T-SEARCH long-term analysis. J Am Coll Cardiol. 2006;47(3):507–14.
2. Kar B, et al. Clinical experience with the TandemHeart percutaneous ventricular assist device. Tex Heart Inst J. 2006;33(2):111–5.
3. Kar B, et al. Hemodynamic support with a percutaneous left ventricular assist device during stenting of an unprotected left main coronary artery. Tex Heart Inst J. 2004;31(1):84–6.
4. Babaev A, et al. Trends in management and outcomes of patients with acute myocardial infarction complicated by cardiogenic shock. JAMA. 2005;294(4):448–54.
5. Laschinger JC, et al. 'Pulsatile' left atrial-femoral artery bypass. A new method of preventing extension of myocardial infarction. Arch Surg. 1983;118(8):965–9.
6. Laschinger JC, et al. Adjunctive left ventricular unloading during myocardial reperfusion plays a major role in minimizing myocardial infarct size. J Thorac Cardiovasc Surg. 1985;90(1):80–5.
7. Catinella FP, et al. Left atrium-to-femoral artery bypass: effectiveness in reduction of acute experimental myocardial infarction. J Thorac Cardiovasc Surg. 1983;86(6):887–96.
8. Cheng JM, et al. Percutaneous left ventricular assist devices vs. intra-aortic balloon pump counterpulsation for treatment of cardiogenic shock: a meta-analysis of controlled trials. Eur Heart J. 2009;30(17):2102–8.

Aortic Valve Interventions: Balloon Aortic Valvuloplasty/Transcatheter Aortic Valve Replacement

26

Surabhi Madhwal, Anitha Rajamanickam, and Annapoorna Kini

This chapter explains steps of aortic valvuloplasty and transcatheter aortic valve replacement.

Balloon Aortic Valvuloplasty (BAV) (Fig. 26.1)

General Overview

Indications See Table 26.1

Contraindications

Absolute: Severe aortic regurgitation (AI)
Relative: Moderate AI

Equipment

- Sheaths:
  - Definite BAV: Single arterial access
    Micropuncture access kit: 6-, 7.5-, 8-, 11-/12-/13-French (Fr) sheaths (depending on the balloon size)
  - For possible BAV: Single arterial access
    Micropuncture access kit: 6- and 7.5-Fr sheaths

S. Madhwal, MD • A. Rajamanickam, MD • A. Kini, MD, MRCP, FACC (✉)
Department of Interventional Cardiology, Mount Sinai Hospital,
One Gustave Levy Place, Madison Avenue, New York, NY 10029, USA
e-mail: Surabhi.medhwal@mountsinai.org, madhwas@gmail.com; arajamanickam@gmail.com,
Anitha.Rajamanickam@mountsinai.org; Annapoorna.kini@mountsinai.org

© Springer-Verlag London 2014
A. Kini et al. (eds.), *Practical Manual of Interventional Cardiology*,
DOI 10.1007/978-1-4471-6581-1_26

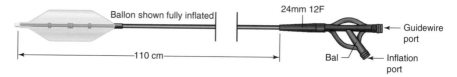

Fig. 26.1 BAV balloon

Table 26.1 BAV in adults >21 years of age with severe aortic stenosis

Indication	Class
Bridge to aortic valve replacement in hemodynamically unstable patients	IIa
Palliation in patients with serious comorbid conditions who are deemed high risk for aortic valve replacement	IIb
Prior to urgent noncardiac surgery	IIb
Before TAVR as a bridge to the procedure	IIb
Alternative to AVR	III

- Catheters:
  - Swan-Ganz catheter
  - 5-Fr Amplatz right 2 (AR2)
  - 6-Fr Judkins left 4 (JL4)
- Wires:
  - 0.035″ standard J-wire
  - 0.038″ straight-tip stiff Terumo® wire
  - 0.035″ Amplatz Super Stiff™ wire (Fig. 26.2)
- Balloon:
  - Z-MED II™ balloon (18–23 mm)
  - True™ balloon (20–22)
- Closure device:
  - Perclose×2 for definite BAV (need only 1 for possible BAV)
- Other equipments:
  - Contrast 50 cc, diluted 1:3
  - 3 manifolds
  - Heparin 2000 units prior to crossing the valve and Angiomax 1/2 bolus (0.375 mg/kg) after the valve is crossed in preparation for the BAV
  - Atropine or neosynephrine if needed to maintain an adequate heart rate and blood pressure
  - Temporary venous pacemaker (TVP)

Vascular access

- Definite BAV:
  - Single arterial access
    - 6-Fr sheath in common femoral artery (use micropuncture to ensure that enrty site is in the CFA and the groin can be sutured with a Perclose device).
    - Place two suture-based closure device (Perclose) in orthogonal positions (referred as Preclose). After Preclose, upgrade to an 8 Fr sheath.

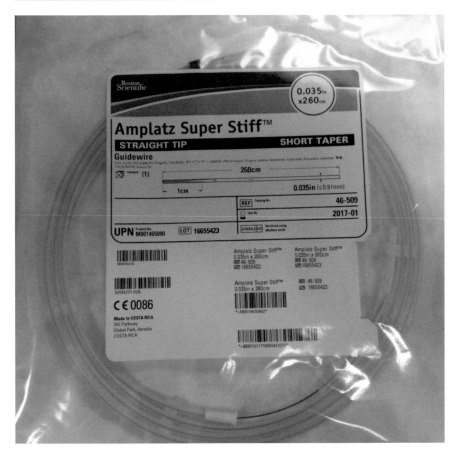

Fig. 26.2 Straight-tip Amplatz Super Stiff™ wire

- Venous access: Femoral vein with 7.5 Fr sheath for hemodynamic assessment using a Swan-Ganz catheter.
- **Possible BAV:**
  - Single arterial access:
    - 6-Fr sheath in common femoral artery (use micropuncture to ensure that enrty site is in the CFA and the groin can be sutured with a Perclose device).
    - Place one suture-based closure device (Perclose) in the same direction as the needle puncture (referred as Preclose). After Preclose, upgrade to an 8 Fr sheath (see Chap. 13).

  Venous access: Femoral vein (7.5 Fr sheath) for Swan-Ganz hemodynamic assessment.

Angiographic views

Aortogram: LAO 30°

Crossing the valve: LAO 30°

Inflation of balloon: RAO 30°

Crossing of the aortic valve

• *Catheter manipulation*
  – Advance Amplatz right 2 (AR2) or Amplatz left 1 (AL1) catheter to the aortic root. Amplatz left 2 (AL2) can be used for very large aortic root, and AR1 and JR4 for small root occasionally, an MP catheter may be required.
  – Once catheter is positioned in the aorta, compare the pressure in the aorta to the femoral side-arm pressure (both transducers need to be zeroed and flushed again). Measure the difference Ao-FA gradient between the central aortic pressure and common femoral arterial pressure Ao-FA. If the difference is more than 10 mm Hg, a double-lumen pigtail should be used.
  – In 30° LAO view, perform a root aortogram and store this image as a reference picture on the second monitor. Pull the catheter back with a slow but firm clockwise rotation to direct the catheter tip to the center of the valve plane.
  – Cross the aortic valve with a 0.038″ straight-tip hydrophilic guidewire (Terumo®).
• *Wire manipulation*
  – In the same fluoroscopic view as the reference image, move the guide wire with firm gentle movements in and out of the catheter tip with the right hand, while the left hand torques the catheter to keep in plane the valve orifice.
  – Once the wire crosses the aortic valve, it is advanced to the middle of the LV, and the fluoroscopic view is changed to RAO to see the wire tip
  – The catheter is then advanced over the guidewire and positioned in mid-ventricular position in RAO 30° view.
  – Connect the catheter to the manifold system and check the left ventricle-femoral artery gradient (LV-FA). If original femoral pressures were discrepant by more than 10 mmHg with the aortic pressure, then double-lumen pigtail (Langston) catheter is placed with exchange length J wire into ventricle. If the central aortic pressure was greater than the FA pressure, subtract the Ao-FA value from the gradient measured across the valve to get the true gradient across the valve. If the central aortic pressure was lesser than the FA pressure, add the Ao-FA value from the gradient measured across the valve to get the true gradient across the valve.
  – Use dobutamine for low-gradient, low-flow aortic stenosis (AS) if left ventricular ejection fraction (LVEF) is <50 % as per protocol
  – If valvuloplasty is appropriate, then advance Amplatz Super Stiff™ wire (J loop at the end and secondary curve at 5 cm proximally, Fig. 26.3) in LV, through the AR2/Langston catheter.

Balloon management

• *Balloon sizing*:
  – Around 1:0.9 to annulus size.
  – NuMED Z-MED II™ balloon catheter: 20 mm (11 Fr sheath), 22 mm (12 Fr sheath), 23 mm (13 Fr sheath) and 25 mm (14 Fr sheath)
  – Use the smaller 20 mm balloon if the valve is densely calcified or the aortic annulus is small (<19 mm by echocardiography).

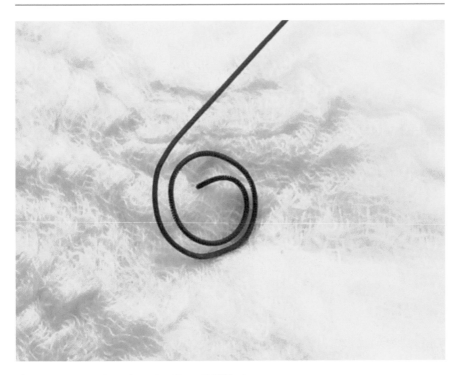

Fig. 26.3 The shaping of Amplatz Super Stiff™ wire

- In general, we begin with a 22-mm Z-MED II™ balloon. In most of our cases, we do not use a larger balloon, though a 25-mm balloon can be used if the aortic annulus diameter is larger than 24 mm.
- True™ balloon: 20 mm (11-Fr sheath) and 22 mm (12-Fr sheath).
- Pediatric Atlas balloon 20 mm (9-Fr sheath) and Tyshak 22-mm balloon (8-Fr sheath).
- *Balloon Preparation*
  - Flush the balloon through the flush port. Attach the 3-way stopcock to the balloon inflation extension of the catheter. Attach a 60-cc syringe filled with a 40 cc of diluted contrast (1:3) to the straight port of the stopcock. De-air the balloon by pulling negative with a 60-cc syringe. Repeat three to four times to ensure the balloon does not have air (Fig. 26.1) and remove air from the syringe as well. Attach a another 10 cc balloon filled with contrast/saline (diluted 1:3) to the other port.

Temporary pacemaker use

- Position a balloon tipped temporary pacemaker in the right ventricular apex/posterior wall through the femoral vein after removing the Swan-Ganz catheter and deflate the temporary wire tip balloon to secure the position. The pulse generator has a capability of up to 220 beats/min.

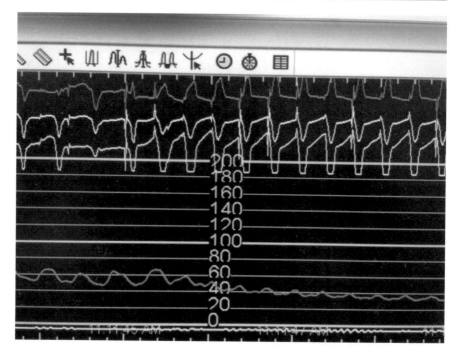

Fig. 26.4 Rapid pacing at 180 beats/min with drop in systolic pressure to 50 mmHg

- Capture is verified prior to balloon inflation (test at least 10–20 beats/min faster than the intrinsic rhythm). Use the pulse generator to pace at 180 beats/min (or above) to decrease systolic blood pressure to 50 mmHg. If BP does not decrease, or 2:1 conduction block is seen, a slower rate may be considered (160/min) (see Fig. 26.4).

Balloon inflation

- While pacing, exert simultaneous forward pressure on the balloon catheter (loaded on the stiff wire). Inflate the balloon via 60-cc syringe and via 10-cc syringe if needed to ensure complete expansion. Look for loss of aortic pressure waveform with balloon inflation and disappearance of waist at valve orifice (see Fig. 26.5). In case the BAV is done as a part of a transcatheter valve replacement, a 20-cc aortogram may be performed (20-cc volume with flow rate of 20 cc/s at 700 psi) to look for adequacy of balloon size.

Balloon deflation

- Immediately after balloon inflation and complete expansion, deflate the balloon by applying negative 60-cc syringe and while maintaining negative pressure pull the rapidly deflating balloon into the ascending aorta and wait for restoration of aortic waveform (for CABG cases pull the balloon in the descending aorta to avoid graft compromise). If hypotension or bradycardia persists, then administer phenylephrine

Fig. 26.5 Valvuloplasty

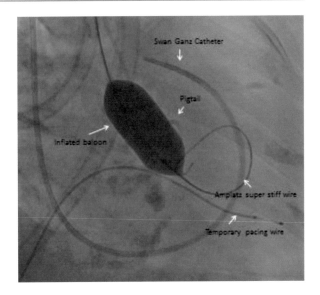

and atropine as needed and be vigilant of other causes of hypotension (tamponade, aortic dissection, rupture retroperitoneal bleed). Pull the balloon out with negative pressure on the 60-cc syringe usually through the arterial sheath. If the balloon gets stuck in the sheath, then take the balloon and sheath out while maintaining the wire in LV under fluoroscopy and replace with a new sheath over the wire.

Post-procedure assessment

- Recheck the transvalvular pressure gradient with AR2 catheter in LV and side port of femoral arterial sheath (peak to peak). If the gradient is reduced by 2/3 of the initial gradient or the valve area doubles, then the procedure is considered successful. If not, then repeat the procedure with a larger balloon.
- Pull AR2 catheter in the aorta and perform aortogram in LAO 30 projection to evaluate the aortic regurgitation post BAV.
- Remove the temporary pacemaker (TPM), and reintroduce the PA catheter to measure PA, PCWP, and CO.

Complications

- Differential causes of hypotension (including access-related hemorrhage, tamponade, LV rupture, and aortic dissection)
- Acute aortic regurgitation

Sheath removal

- Arterial access is closed with 2 preclose stitches (see Chap. 13)

Post-procedure management and monitoring CCU care

TAVR

Edwards SAPIEN valve is a balloon expandable platform, and it is currently available in the USA in three sizes, 23, 26 and 29 mm in diameter (Fig. 26.6).

Valve preparation

- The valve is prepared and mounted onto a sheath system for implantation on the back table (Fig. 26.7a, b).
- The valve is mounted on the de-aired balloon and then crimped to fit in the sheath delivery system (Fig. 26.8a, b).
- The valve is ready to enter to sheath delivery system (Fig. 26.13); the cone is positioned according to the orientation of the valve. The suture line bears a colored indicator that should be closer to LV side. This is verified with the implanting physician (Fig. 26.9a, b).

Access preparation for transfemoral approach

- The femoral arterial access is serially dilated to accommodate sheaths, or dynamic expansion mechanism is used which allows for transient sheath expansion during transcatheter valve delivery (Fig. 26.10). A 16-French sheath (for 23-mm SAPIEN XT valve), 18-French sheath (for 26 mm SAPIEN XT valve), and 20 French sheath (for 26-mm SAPIEN XT valve) are used. The sheath is advanced under fluoroscopic guidance over a stiff long wire.

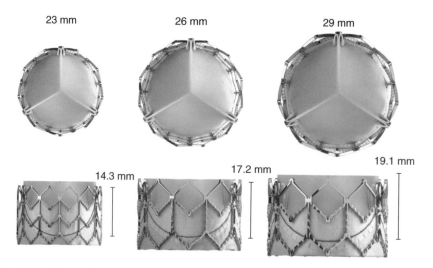

Fig. 26.6 Edward SAPIEN valve (© Edwards Lifesciences LLC, Irvine, CA. All rights reserved. Used with the permission of Edwards Lifesciences LLC)

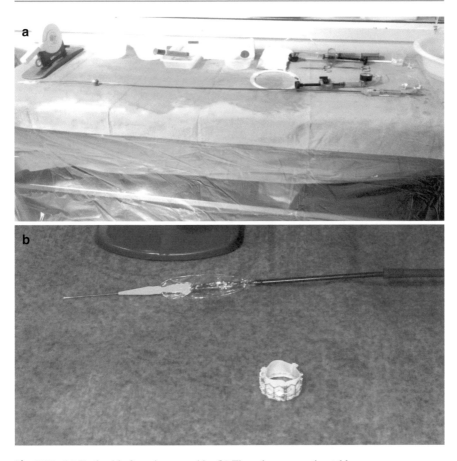

Fig. 26.7 (**a**) Back table for valve assembly. (**b**) The valve preparation table

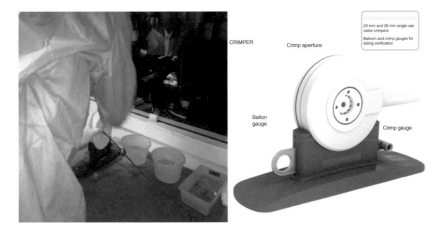

Fig. 26.8 Valve being crimped for delivery (© Edwards Lifesciences LLC, Irvine, CA. All rights reserved. Used with the permission of Edwards Lifesciences LLC)

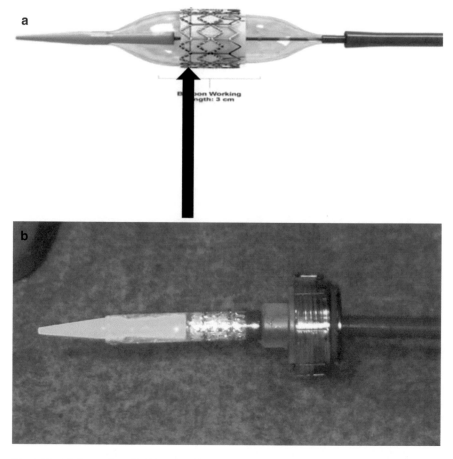

Fig. 26.9 (a) Suture line (© Edwards Lifesciences LLC, Irvine, CA. All rights reserved. Used with the permission of Edwards Lifesciences LLC). (b) Valve is mounted on delivery system

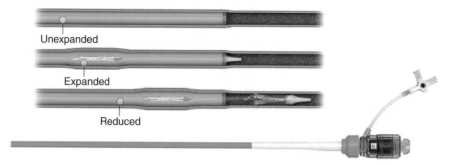

Fig. 26.10 Dilator kit for access management with Edwards expandable introducer sheath set (eSheath) (© Edwards Lifesciences LLC, Irvine, CA. All rights reserved. Used with the permission of Edwards Lifesciences LLC)

Implantation angle

- The implantation angle is the fluoroscopic angle where the bases of all three cusps are aligned in one line. Annular plane is an imaginary plane that touches the lowest points of all 3 cusps (Fig. 26.11).
- Figure 26.12 shows an aortogram: A 5 Fr angled pigtail is placed in the noncoronary cusp, and aortogram is performed identifying a projection with all three cusps visible (a careful review of CT scan reconstructions can help identify the best fluoroscopic view to get the appropriate annular planes).

Advancement of the valve

- The balloon-mounted valve is then advanced to the aortic valve position using angiographic and echocardiographic guidance. For ease of prosthesis arch transit, the delivery platform is equipped with the NovaFlex system which should be mostly fully flexed upon entering the distal aortic arch (Fig. 26.13).

Crossing the aortic valve with Edwards SAPIEN delivery system

- Before crossing the aortic arch, the delivery catheter is flexed, a left anterior oblique projection is obtained, and the catheter is advanced with traction maintained on the wire. When the nose cone is past the aortic valve, return to the prior fluoroscopic view for implantation of the valve. It is important that the wire position in the ventricle is maintained at all times even when difficulty is encountered

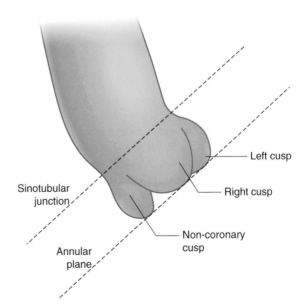

Fig. 26.11 Annular plane is an imaginary line joining the lower part of 3 cusps

Fig. 26.12 Angiographic
view of annular plane

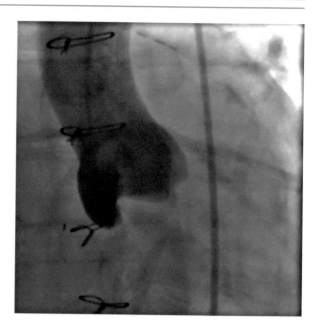

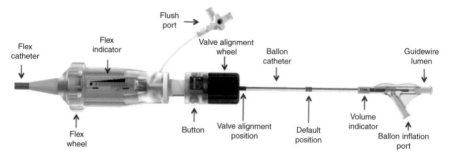

Fig. 26.13 NovaFlex delivery system for Edward SAPIEN valve (© Edwards Lifesciences LLC, Irvine, CA. All rights reserved. Used with the permission of Edwards Lifesciences LLC)

advancing the catheter system through the stenotic native valve (as this valve cannot be retracted in the sheath and it is very unlikely that a new wire will cross the valve through the valve delivery system).

- Once the bioprosthesis crosses the native valve, the outer "flex" catheter is withdrawn so as not to interfere with balloon inflation (there is a fluoroscopically visible marker).

Edwards SAPIEN delivery system

- For the transfemoral approach, the recommended positioning of the prosthesis is 60–40 %, which means 60 % of the prosthesis should be on the ventricular side

Fig. 26.14 Positioning of valve

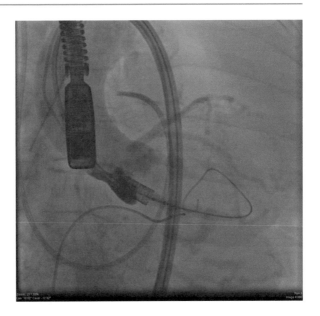

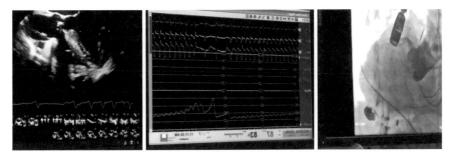

Fig. 26.15 After confirmation of the valve position on echocardiogram and angiogram, pacing is started on command of the operator, and blood pressure is depressed to systolic 50 mm of Hg

of the aortic annulus with 40 % of the prosthesis on the aortic side of the annulus. For thoracic approach 50–50 % is preferable (Fig. 26.14).

- The valve plane is confirmed with the pigtail placed on the noncoronary native cusp and injections through this catheter assist in valve placement (Fig. 26.12). The correct orientation of the prosthesis should be confirmed both visually prior to placement into the introducer sheath and angiographically prior to deployment (during a test v-pace run) (Fig. 26.14).
- The primary operator defines the roles of the assistants (the "inflator," the "contrast injector," and the "pacer"). Next, transvalvular flow is severely depressed by rapid ventricular pacing (Fig. 26.15).
- The primary operator gives simple, clear instructions for pacing, and when blood pressure drops to around 50 mm of Hg, the valve is then balloon expanded in position with rapid but steady inflation mode. The primary operator calls out

Fig. 26.16 Edwards
SAPIEN valve being
deployed

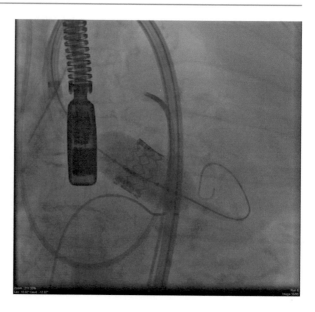

1–1,000, 2–1,000, 3–1,000, 4–1,000, 5–1,000, 6–1,000 to ensure proper expansion of the valve (Figs. 26.15 and 26.16). The rapid pacing can be stopped by the implanting physician by giving clear instructions to "stop pacing." The balloon is deflated and pulled in the ascending aorta. Be well prepared to manage complications expediently. If there is moderate to severe aortic insufficiency from a paravalvular leak after the deployment, post-dilation may need to be performed by adding 1 cc of the dye to increase the capacity of the balloon to a larger size.

CoreValve deployment performed using a 18-Fr sheath. The percutaneous closure is planned at the time of getting access with perclose suture device (Abbott Vascular, Abbot Park, IL). Prior to implantation of the prosthesis, aortic angiography is performed. Subsequently aortic valvuloplasty is done (as described above). A 26-, 29-, or 31-mm prosthesis is implanted for aortic annulus diameter of 20–23 mm, 24–27 mm, and 27–29 mm respectively.

- The valve is prepared by washing the valve apparatus in a ice cold saline bath, soaking the nitinol frame in a cold saline bath, and loading the valve into the 18 Fr introducer sheaths all of which require ice cold temperatures. The low temperature causes the ninitol frame to become more flexible and compressible into the small delivery catheter (Fig. 26.17a–c).
- Delivery system should be placed the way it should face during the advancement through the aorta (Fig. 26.18a, b).
- The CoreValve is loaded over the Amplatz Super Stiff™ wire, and the valve is initially within the annulus level positioned between first and second ring at the annular level. There is a 4-mm distance between two rings (Fig. 26.19a–c).

Fig. 26.17 (a) CoreValve
being assembled. (b)
CoreValve being
assembled. (c) CoreValve
being assembled

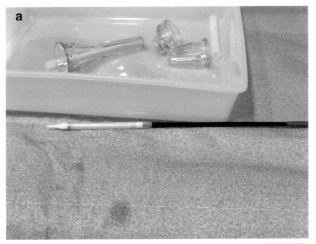

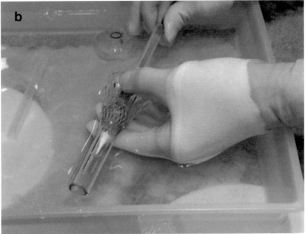

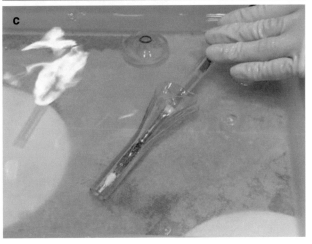

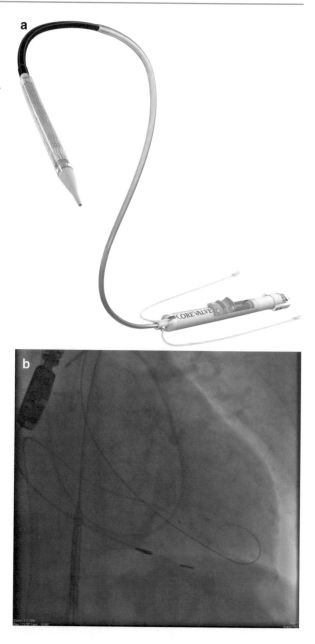

Fig. 26.18 (a) CoreValve delivery system (© Medtronic, Inc. All rights reserved. Used with the permission of Medtronic, Inc.). (b) CoreValve delivery system being advanced

- The CoreValve is positioned 4-mm deep (about 0.5 diamond or one ring below the annulus which is the lowest part of the visualized right coronary cusp by pigtail injection, Figure 26.19b, c). The fluoroscopic view for valve implantation is guided by the radioopaque marker on the prosthesis; it should appear as a straight line (Fig. 26.20a); if it appears as an oval ring (Fig. 26.20b), adjust fluoroscopic view (usually caudal) to make it appear as a single line.

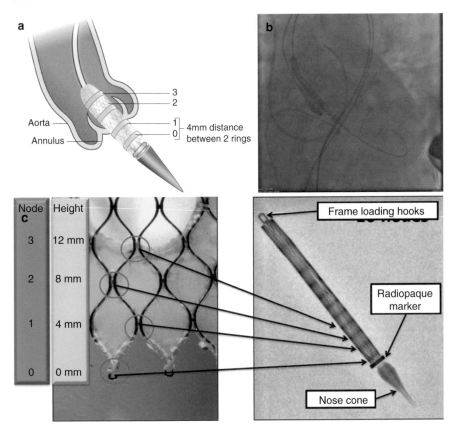

Fig. 26.19 (**a**) CoreValve being positioned between ring 1 and 2 which is proximally 4–8 mm (© Medtronic, Inc. All rights reserved. Used with the permission of Medtronic, Inc.). (**b**) CoreValve being positioned between rings 1 and 2 which is proximally 4–8 mm. (**c**) Fluoroscopic correlate of CoreValve (© Medtronic, Inc. All rights reserved. Used with the permission of Medtronic, Inc.)

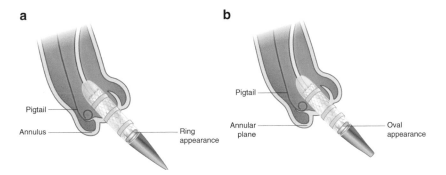

Fig. 26.20 (**a**) Ring appearance (© Medtronic, Inc. All rights reserved. Used with the permission of Medtronic, Inc.). (**b**) Oval appearance (© Medtronic, Inc. All rights reserved. Used with the permission of Medtronic, Inc.)

- Once the markers are aligned and the valve is at least 0.5 diamond space below the annulus, the second operator will start releasing the valve with a clockwise motion of the knob (Fig. 26.21). About 20 turns are required to reach the initial position.
- Continuously monitor under fluoroscopy. The valve can still be adjusted as long as it has not touched the annulus. After annular contact, valve can still be pulled back but cannot be pushed back in safely (Fig. 26.22).
- If the angle of the LV/aorta is large, an eccentric position will be assumed and the valve may be released deeper than usual (1 diamond = 8 mm below the annulus) to avoid the malapposition at one side and dislodgement of the valve above the annulus level.
- Assess the position of the bioprosthesis with the pigtail in noncoronary cusp. After checking that the valve is not too deep, it can be released. Once release is started it should be slow till it is flared to the annulus level (Fig. 26.22). Once the flared valve has touched the annulus, the rest of the valve can be deployed under moderate pacing

Fig. 26.21 The valve with clockwise motion of the knob

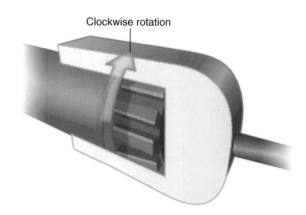

Clockwise rotation

Fig. 26.22 After annular contact, valve can repositioned by pulling up

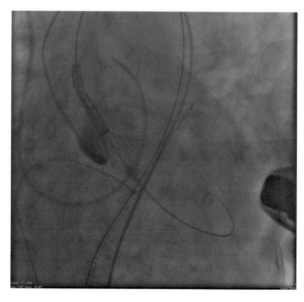

(100–120/min) until 2/3 of the valve is released. At this point the valve is fully functional, and blood pressure should be stabilized (Fig. 26.23). If pigtail injection shows the valve is too deep before full release, it can be pulled back carefully by primary operator with constant heavy pressure on the valve or pulling on the Amplatz Super Stiff™ wire (while ensuring that the Amplatz Super Dtiff wire is always in the LV). The pigtail is pulled to the arch. After deployment of the valve, the tension on delivery system is checked: if the system is touching the lower wall of the transverse aorta, then the tension is released by pushing forward and then the valve is completely released by clocking the knob, and delivery system is withdrawn while maintaining the wire position in LV. The pigtail is advanced in the LV to measure the LV-Ao gradient.

- The delivery system is taken out by sheathing the remaining frame by advancing the knob and rotating the back end. Once the valve is fully released and if all the points are still not detached (verified in two fluoroscopic views), then rotate catheter with a firm push to a 270°; if there is no effect, then rotate in the opposite direction for another 270° (Fig. 26.24a, b).

Fig. 26.23 Optimum position around half diamond below annular plane (© Medtronic, Inc. All rights reserved. Used with the permission of Medtronic, Inc.)

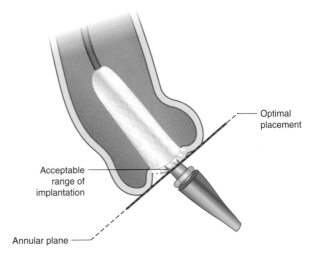

Fig. 26.24 (a) Valve being released. (b) Turning 270° to release the valve

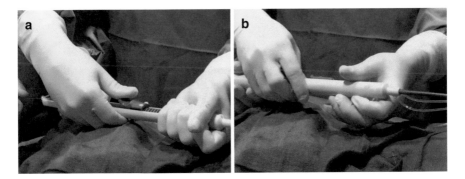

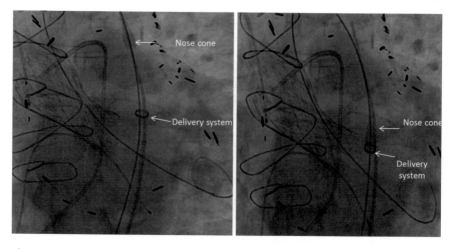

Fig. 26.25 Nose cone and delivery system are together before withdrawal of the system

- At the descending aorta, fluoroscopic confirmation is done ensuring nose cone and delivery system is together and the knob is at the front end (Fig. 26.25). Then the delivery system is taken out of the body.
- The procedure is finished with aortogram to assess for aortic regurgitation.

Troubleshooting techniques

- If valve is too deep after full deployment of the valve, it may be snared to higher position.
- If leak still persists, a second valve can be placed in appropriate position.
- If the valve is deployed above the annulus after it is fully released, then it is critical to maintain wire position in the LV and implant a second valve in an appropriate (lower position) at the annulus level.
- If there is severe paravalvular leak without a deep (low) position of the valve, post dilation with a balloon size 1:1 to the maximum annular diameter should be performed.

Percutaneous Mitral Balloon Valvotomy

27

Sadik Raja Panwar, Anitha Rajamanickam, and Annapoorna Kini

Mitral stenosis (MS) is a progressive disabling disease for which till 1984 open surgery was the only cure. Introduction of percutaneous mitral balloon valvotomy (PMBV) by Inoue in 1984 for the treatment of selected MS patients has transformed the treatment of MS.

Indications

AHA/ACC guidelines for indications of PBMV is listed in Table 27.1 [1].

A successful result can be predicted by a Wilkins score of ≤ 8, which is calculated by assigning a point of 0 to 4 for each of the following four criteria for a maximum score of 16 [2].

- Leaflet mobility
- Leaflet thickening
- Leaflet calcification
- Subvalvular thickening

S.R. Panwar, MD • A. Rajamanickam, MD • A. Kini, MD, MRCP, FACC (✉)
Department of Interventional Cardiology, Mount Sinai Hospital,
One Gustave Levy Place, Madison Avenue, New York, NY 10029, USA
e-mail: drsrpanwar@gmail.com; arajamanickam@gmail.com,
Anitha.Rajamanickam@mountsinai.org; Annapoorna.kini@mountsinai.org

© Springer-Verlag London 2014
A. Kini et al. (eds.), *Practical Manual of Interventional Cardiology*,
DOI 10.1007/978-1-4471-6581-1_27

Table 27.1 Indications for percutaneous balloon mitral valvulopasty (PBMV) as per guidelines

Favorable valve morphology in the absence of contraindications	
Symptomatic patients with severe MS (MVA <1.5 cm²)ᵃ	Ia
Asymptomatic patients with very severe MS (MVA ≤1.0 cm²)ᵃ	IIa
Asymptomatic patients with severe MS (MVA ≤1.5 cm²)ᵃ who have new onset of AF	IIb
Symptomatic patients with MVA >1.5 cm² if there is evidence of hemodynamically significant MS during exercise [PASP >60 mmHg, PCWP >25 mmHg, mean valve gradient >15 mmHg]	
Considered for severely symptomatic patients with severe MS (MVA ≤1.5 cm²) who have suboptimal valve anatomy and are not candidates for surgery or at high risk for surgery	

ᵃFavorable valve morphology (Wilkins score <8) in the absence of contraindications

Contraindications to Percutaneous Balloon Mitral Valvuloplasty (PBMV)

Persistent left atrial or left atrial appendage thrombus
More than moderate mitral regurgitation
Massive or bicommissural calcification
Severe concomitant aortic valve disease
Severe organic tricuspid stenosis or severe functional regurgitation with enlarged
    annulus
Severe concomitant coronary artery disease requiring bypass surgery

Preparation

- Labs: CBC, BMP, and coagulation profile
- Trans-esophageal echocardiography (TEE): To exclude LAA/LA thrombus and to calculate the Wilkins score.

Equipment

Sheaths For definite BMV – 8 Fr sheath for right venous access, 7.5 Fr sheath for left venous access, 5 Fr sheath for left arterial access and a 14 Fr Mullins sheath
    For possible BMV – 7.5 Fr sheath for left venous access and a 5 Fr sheath for left arterial access

Catheters Swan-Ganz catheter, 5-Fr pigtail catheter, and Brockenbrough needle

Wires 0.035″ standard J-wire, 0.032″ straight wire, and 0.025 Swan wire

Balloon

- Inoue balloon kit (balloon size is calculated in mm = [Height of patient in cm/10] + 10)
- 0.025 curled guidewire
- 14-Fr dilator
- Preshaped stylet (LV wire)

Contrast 50 cc (no dilution)

Manifolds Three manifolds

Heparin 10,000 IU/10 cc

Vascular Access for Definite BMV 8 Fr right FV, 7.5 Fr left femoral vein, and 5 Fr left femoral artery

Vascular Access for Possible BMV 7.5 Fr left femoral vein and 5 Fr left femoral artery

Procedural Steps

- Assess coronary anatomy for patient >40 years of age.
- Perform a complete right heart catheterization first through the left femoral vein.
- Leave the Swan-Ganz catheter in PA for hemodynamic monitoring during the procedure.
- Advance 5-Fr pigtail catheter over J-wire to LV via left FA access and wedge the Swan-Ganz catheter. Record the left ventricular end diastolic pressure (LVEDP) and pulmonary capillary wedge pressure (PCWP) simultaneously for the transmitral gradient and calculate the mitral valve area (MVA).
- Medrad LV gram (30 cc volume at 20 cc/s at 450 PSI in LAO 45 and RAO 15 positions to evaluate for mitral regurgitation (MR)).
- Pull pigtail into ascending aorta and perform an aortogram in LAO 30 to assess for coexisting AI.
- Place the pigtail in the aorta in noncoronary cusp.

Transseptal Puncture

- In AP position, advance 0.032 wire to SVC via right FV and change to 8-Fr Mullins sheath.
- Remove 0.032 wire and Mullins sheath dilator and de-air the system.
- Advance Brockenbrough needle (with third transducer attached) through Mullins sheath and keep the tip of the needle 2 cm below the tip of the Mullins sheath.

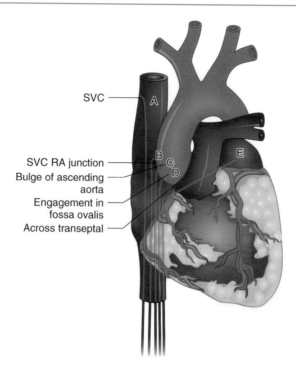

Fig. 27.1 Landmarks of descent for transseptal puncture AP view. (*A*) SVC. (*B*) SVC-RA junction. (*C*) Bulge of ascending aorta. (*D*) Engagement in fossa ovalis. (*E*) Across transseptal puncture

- Use AP view to confirm the correct needle position and pull down the sheath and needle as one unit. Position the Mullins sheath in RA against the interatrial septum (IAS) in AP position.
- Maintain needle tip direction indicator (at the needle hub) at 5'o clock position.
- In the AP position, while keeping the needle inside the sheath, position the needle tip by clockwise rotation to the optimal IAS puncture site (clockwise rotation moves the needle tip toward posterior edge of LA, anticlockwise rotation toward aorta).
- At the midpoint of "end on mitral annulus" (in AP) and midpoint of anterior and posterior halves of IAS (in LAO), penetrate IAS. Note LA pressure tracing and aspirate bright oxygenated blood to check for oxygen saturation and/or inject contrast through needle to confirm location.
- Advance the needle (~2 cm) into LA and advance Mullins sheath over the needle while holding it firmly.
  - *See* Figs. 27.1 and 27.2a–e *landmarks of descent for transseptal puncture.*
- Withdraw the needle and aspirate blood to check for oxygen saturation.
- Give 10,000 IU of heparin once IA is crossed (or 100 U/kg).
- Measure transmitral gradient using LV pigtail catheter and Mullins sheath.
  - Figures 27.3a, b proper orientation for septal puncture.

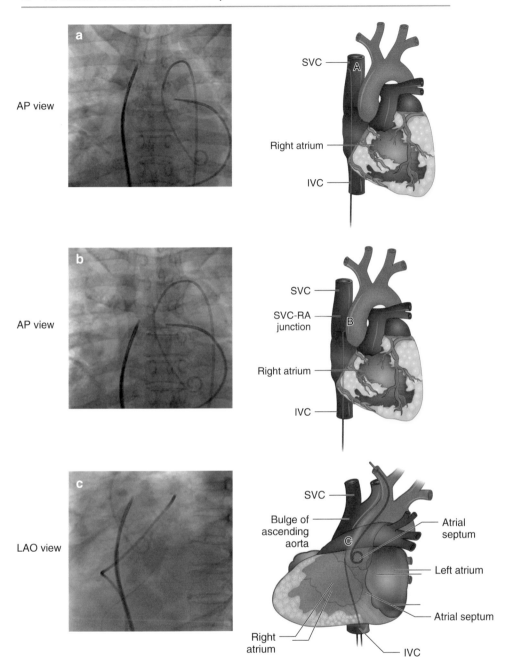

Fig. 27.2 (**a–e**) Landmarks of descent for transseptal puncture with fluoroscopy pictures. (**a**) AP view. (**b**) AP view. (**c**) LAO view. (**d**) LAO view. (**e**) LAO view

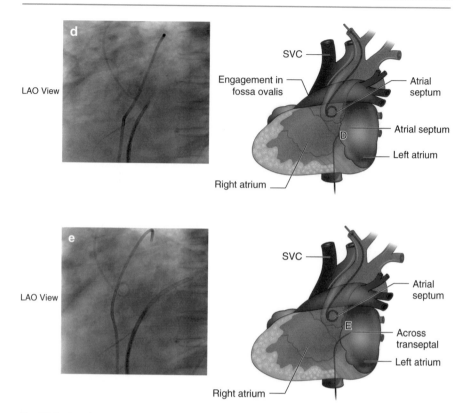

Fig. 27.2 (continued)

Balloon Preparation

- Open the vent port (short port) and flush the balloon with undiluted contrast.
- Attach the contrast-filled marked syringe to inflation port (longer port).
- Inflate the balloon to correct size and measure with measurement gauge. Inject dye through vent port if balloon is to be upsized.
- Insert the metal balloon stretching tube in the center lumen and lock it into place (metal to metal attachment).

Balloon Insertion and Crossing the Mitral Valve

- With the Mullins sheath in LA, now introduce 0.025 curled guidewire into LA and allow it to coil with top of the coil against roof of LA.
- After removing the Mullins sheath, introduce 14-Fr dilator over the guidewire into LA across IAS puncture site.
- The stretched balloon is now inserted along the 0.025 curled guidewire to the top of the curve. At this point, the stretching tube is released (loosen metal-to-plastic connection) and withdrawn 2–3 cm and advanced further into LA following the

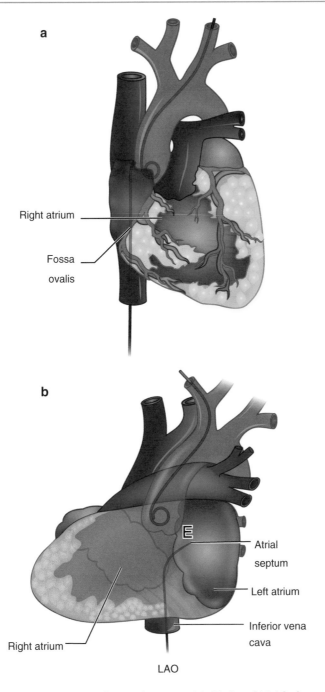

Fig. 27.3 (**a**, **b**) Proper orientation for septal puncture. (**a**) AP view. (**b**) LAO view

curve of the wire. Thereafter unfasten the metal-to-metal connection and remove the stretching tube completely at this point.

- Now remove the 0.025 curled guidewire while maintaining balloon position on LA.
- Insert the stylet through center lumen and guide the balloon into LV in RAO view (counterclockwise rotation of the stylet with gentle withdrawal of the balloon).
- Once the balloon is across the MV orifice, observe free movement toward the apex.
- Withdraw the balloon partially and push volume into the balloon until the distal end inflates.
- Maintain gentle traction and rest the balloon against the mitral orifice.
- Inflate the balloon fully once movement toward the LA stops.
- Once the waist disappeared and the balloon is fully inflated to its predetermined size, immediately deflate the balloon and withdraw into LA.
- Using the balloon's central lumen and LV pigtail catheter, measure transmitral gradient.
- Perform Medrad biplane LV gram and compare with pre-procedure LV gram to assess for the worsening of MR. No need for LV gram when the procedure is TEE or ICE (intracardiac echocardiography) guided.
- Document cardiac output (CO), pulmonary artery (PA), and pulmonary capillary wedge (PCW) pressures. If there is no MR and residual mitral gradient >5, repeat the balloon dilation, after increasing the balloon size by 1 cm by injecting the contrast via the vent port.
- Administer intrapulmonary nitro and IV Lasix as necessary.
- Admit patient to coronary intensive care unit (CCU) for observation and restart anticoagulation if indicated.

Complications and Their Management

- Severe MR, which occurs in 2–10 % of patients.
- A large atrial septal defect (greater than 1.5:1 left-to-right shunt) occurs in fewer than 12 % of patients with the double-balloon technique and fewer than 5 % with the Inoue balloon technique. Smaller atrial septal defects may be detected by transesophageal echocardiography in larger numbers of patients.
- Perforation of the left ventricle (0.5–4.0 %).
- Embolic events (0.5–3 %).
- Myocardial infarction (0.3–0.5 %).
- The mortality is 1–2 %, but in carefully selected cases at experienced centers, it is <1 %.

Post-procedure Care and Follow-Up

- As needed by severity of MS and clinical status of the patient. Most patients can be discharged the next day.
- Coumadin if necessary for other reason like atrial fibrillation, to be started or restarted the next day (at least 24 h after the procedure to reduce access site bleeding).

References

1. Nishimura RA, Otto CM, Bonow RO, Carabello BA, Erwin 3rd JP, Guyton RA, O'Gara PT, Ruiz CE, Skubas NJ, Sorajja P, Sundt 3rd TM, Thomas JD. 2014 AHA/ACC guideline for the management of patients with valvular heart disease: a report of the American College of Cardiology/American Heart Association Task Force on practice guidelines. J Am Coll Cardiol. 2014;63(22):e57–e185. doi:10.1016/j.jacc.2014.02.536. Epub 2014 Mar 3. PubMed PMID: 24603191.
2. Wilkins GT, Weyman AE, Abascal VM. Percutaneous balloon dilatation of the mitral valve: an analysis of echocardiographic variables related to outcome and the mechanism of dilatation. Br Heart J. 1988;60(4):299–308.

Alcohol Septal Ablation

28

Rikesh Patel, Anitha Rajamanickam, and Annapoorna Kini

Alcohol septal ablation [ASA] is a percutaneous, minimally invasive procedure performed by interventional cardiologists in carefully selected hypertrophic cardiomyopathy patients who meet strict criteria and are severely symptomatic despite maximal medical therapy. Ablation induces localized myocardial infarction which causes thinning of the basal ventricular septum leading to reduction in dynamic outflow obstruction.

Criteria

- Severe, drug-refractory cardiac symptoms (NYHA/CCS III/IV dyspnea/angina or syncope)
- Dynamic LVOT obstruction (gradient ≥ 50 mmHg at rest or ≥ 50 mmHg with provocation)
- Absence of significant intrinsic mitral valve disease
- Ventricular septal thickness of ≥ 15 mm and systolic anterior motion (SAM) of the mitral valve
- Sufficient basal septal thickness to safely and successfully perform ASA

R. Patel, MD • A. Rajamanickam, MD • A. Kini, MD, MRCP, FACC (✉)
Department of Interventional Cardiology, Mount Sinai Hospital,
One Gustave Levy Place, Madison Avenue, New York, NY 10029, USA
e-mail: rikeshrpatel@gmail.com, rikeshpatel.md@gmail.com;
Annapoorna.kini@mountsinai.org

© Springer-Verlag London 2014
A. Kini et al. (eds.), *Practical Manual of Interventional Cardiology*,
DOI 10.1007/978-1-4471-6581-1_28

Access

- Right common femoral artery (alternatively, radial): 6-Fr sheath
- Left common femoral artery (alternatively radial): 5-Fr sheath
- Right internal jugular vein: temporary pacemaker (if patient does *not* already have a permanent pacemaker (PPM))

Equipment

- 6-Fr sheath and 6-Fr left coronary guide catheter of choice
- 5-Fr multipurpose catheter (MP)
- Temporary pacemaker (with sheath and locking cover)
- 0.014″ guidewire (Fielder™ or Whisper™)
- 100 % absolute alcohol
- Compliant, (OTW) balloon (1.5×9 or 2.0×9 mm)
- Intraprocedural Transthoracic echocardiography (TTE) and definity contrast injection available

Hemodynamic Assessment

- Simultaneous pressure measurement of LV outflow region and ascending aorta (assess for gradient via pullback with MP catheter from LV apex to LV outflow tract).
- Assess for Brockenbrough-Braunwald-Morrow sign (see Fig. 28.1)—drop in post-extrasystolic aortic pulse pressure [1].

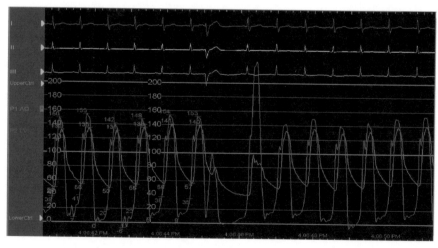

Fig. 28.1 Brockenbrough-Braunwald-Morrow sign

Technique

- Place temporary pacemaker (if no permanent PM) via right internal jugular vein. The temporary pacemaker should be left in place for at least 48 h post ablation.
- Draw baseline CPK, CK-MB, and troponin levels.
- Perform coronary angiography to determine most appropriate septal artery for ablation and to evaluate for CAD.
  - *Both* coronary arteries should be assessed as the proximal RCA can give rise to basal septal arteries.
  - *RAO* (*straight and caudal*) projection: Angulation of origin of septal artery; *cranial* projection: Length of septal and course of septal artery.
- Use MP catheter in LV via second arterial access to measure resting and post-PVC LV gradient.
- Administer Angiomax with goal ACT >300 s.
- 6-Fr guide:
  - Wire the first major septal artery.
  - Negotiate OTW balloon to most basal septal branch.
  - Inflate over-the-wire balloon (size according to septal artery diameter) to 5–6 atm and perform cineangiography of LAD to confirm no compromise of LAD flow and also balloon position.
  - Inject DEFINITY™ contrast (dilute 0.8 mL of DEFINITY into 10 cc saline, then draw up 1 cc into a small syringe and inject 1 cc at a time) while the balloon is inflated. The goal is to avoid enhancement of RV, free walls, or papillary muscles and to delineate the septum. Withdraw the guidewire out of the OTW balloon under water seal.
- Inject absolute alcohol (100 % absolute, 1–3 mL) through the lumen of the inflated balloon (no more than 1 mL/min with a timer). Slow the injections if patient develops heart block, premature ventricular contractions (PVCs), or intraventricular conduction delay (IVCD). Usually, the gradient starts to decline with successful alcohol injection.
- Note: if patient develops transient heart block or IVCD, HOLD injection for 3–5 min (balloon remains inflated) and restart if rhythm reverts to normal. STOP injection if patient has developed persistent heart block or IVCD (even if 1, 2, or 3 cc of alcohol has been injected).
- Continue total balloon inflation time of at least 5 min (after stopping alcohol injection).
- Continue TTE monitoring and measure the LVOT gradient while the balloon is inflated and remove any residual alcohol from lumen by additional saline flush.
- If resting gradient <16 mmHg, deflate balloon and finish after confirming LAD patency.
- If resting LVOT gradient >16 mmHg, consider injecting another septal artery or the same septal artery more proximally [2].
- The average number of arteries injected=1.7; average volume of alcohol injected=3 mL.

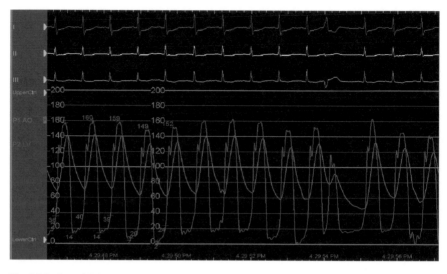

Fig. 28.2 Post-ASA gradients

Post-procedure

- Acute procedural success (80–85 %) is defined as ≥50 % reduction in peak resting or provoked LVOT gradient with a final residual resting gradient of <20 mmHg (see Fig. 28.2).
- Further reduction in LVOT gradient occurs over 3–6 months due to ventricular-remodeling and basal septal thinning.

Complications

- Chest pain during the procedure (This can be usually treated with IV narcotics)
- Most common complication: AV block—10–15 % may require permanent PM; this rate approaches 50 % if baseline LBBB is present of EKG, severe left axis deviation, or wide QRS [3]
- Ventricular fibrillation/tachycardia
- Overall periprocedure mortality of 2 %

Post-procedure

- Observe in ICU setting for at least 2 days. The temporary pacemaker is left in the patient for 48 h post-procedure.

- Post procedural elevation of CPK (between 800 and 1,200 U/L) usually occurs. The amount of elevation depends upon amount of alcohol injected, vessel size, and method of enzyme measurement.
- Patient can be discharged home once CK-MB level is <80 ng/mL.
- Aspirin 81 mg orally daily should be continued indefinitely.
- If a patient is on beta- and/or calcium-channel blockers, medical therapy can be reduced by discontinuation of one class if patient is on both, or reduction in dosage if the patient is only on one class of medication.
- Repeat TTE the next day.
- Follow-up echocardiogram should be performed at 6 months and annually thereafter.

References

1. Braunwald E, Bonow RO. Braunwald's heart disease: a textbook of cardiovascular medicine. 9th ed. Philadelphia: Saunders; 1961, xxiv.
2. Baim DS, Grossman W. Grossman's cardiac catheterization, angiography, and intervention. 7th ed. Philadelphia: Lippincott Williams & Wilkins; 2006. xvii, 807 p. 720–1.
3. El Masry H, Breall JA. Alcohol septal ablation for hypertrophic obstructive cardiomyopathy. Curr Cardiol Rev. 2008;4(3):193–7.

Pericardiocentesis and Balloon Pericardiotomy

29

Rahul Sawant, Anitha Rajamanickam, and Annapoorna Kini

Pericardiocentesis is the percutaneous drainage of fluid from the pericardial space for diagnostic or therapeutic purposes. It is lifesaving in cardiac tamponade. Balloon pericardiotomy is a palliative procedure for the management of recurrent pericardial effusions performed using fluoroscopy and echocardiography as an alternative to surgical pericardial window.

Pericardiocentesis

Indications

- *Emergency*: Cardiac tamponade.
- *Elective*: Diagnosis and therapeutic drainage to alleviate symptoms of pericardial effusion.
- *Relative contraindications*: Aortic dissection, myocardial rupture, bleeding disorder, and traumatic pericardial effusion. For emergency pericardiocentesis in hemodynamically compromised patients, there are no contraindications as withholding treatment results in certain death.

Etiologies

- Metastatic cancer, tuberculosis, and uremia are the most common outpatient etiologies.
- Post-cardiac surgery and iatrogenic following invasive cardiac procedure are the most common inpatient etiologies.

R. Sawant • A. Rajamanickam, MD • A. Kini, MD, MRCP, FACC (✉)
Department of Interventional Cardiology, Mount Sinai Hospital,
One Gustave Levy Place, Madison Avenue, New York, NY 10029, USA
e-mail: drrahulsawant@hotmail.com; arajamanickam@gmail.com,
Anitha.rajamanickam@mountsinai.org; Annapoorna.kini@mountsinai.org

© Springer-Verlag London 2014
A. Kini et al. (eds.), *Practical Manual of Interventional Cardiology*,
DOI 10.1007/978-1-4471-6581-1_29

- Trauma, infection, cardiac failure, collagen vascular disease, mediastinal radiation, and hypothyroidism are some of the other causes of pericardial effusion.

Equipment

- Local anesthetic, pericardial drainage kit which contains 21 and 18 G needles, a 50 ml syringe, a 3-way stop clock, extension tubing, drainage bag, scalpel, puncture needle, 0.35 in. guidewire, dilator, multihole pigtail or straight catheter, 2-0 silk suture, and sterile bottles for sample collection.
- Check coagulation parameters and obtain informed consent for an elective procedure.
- Fluoroscopy-guided pericardiocentesis with or without echo is recommended. In life-threatening situations, it can be done at the bedside in the ER or CCU preferably under echocardiographic guidance.

Procedure

- Place patient on the cath lab table or bed supine position. A 30-40° elevation of the head of the bed is also recommended as this position brings the pericardial space closer to the anterior chest wall and the fluid collects inferiorly and posteriorly.
- Clean and drape the operative area using aseptic precautions. Inject a generous amount local anesthesia in the area about an inch below and lateral to the xiphoid process.
- In unstable cardiac tamponade, start and avoid sedation.

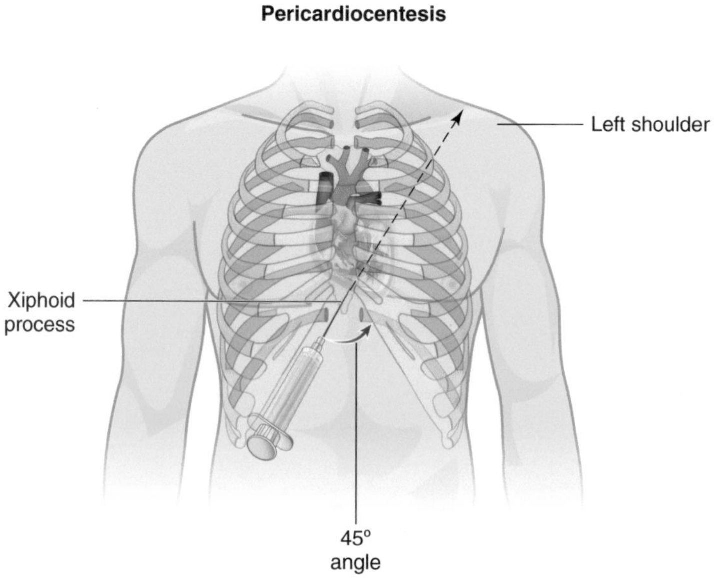

Pericardiocentesis

Fig. 29.1 Site of entry

- Usually approach is a subxiphoid access. Echocardiograhy helps identify the distance of the effusion from the skin and if other entry sites are required. Entry occurs usually 1–2 cm lateral and below the xiphoid process. Make a small skin incision with the #11 scalpel (Fig. 29.1).
- In our practice, we use a 15 cm 18 G needle with a mandrel. Advance the needle with the mandrel in place at 90° angle to the skin for 2–3 cm. Then direct it upward toward the left midclavicle under echo guidance. As the needle enters the pericardium, a giveaway sensation is felt. The mandrel is removed and a 10 cc syringe is attached, maintaining negative suction.
- Once the fluid is aspirated in the syringe, confirm needle position using echocardiography. Some recommend injecting agitated saline in the pericardial space and confirm needle position by the echocardiographic presence of micro-bubbles in the pericardial cavity. Advance a 0.035 wire into the pericardial space.
- Confirm the posterior course of the wire in the LAO view. If fluoroscopy shows the wire curling around the heart border toward the root and the presence of wire in the pericardial space is confirmed.
- After confirming that the wire is in the pericardial space, remove the needle leaving the 0.035 wire in place. Advance a dilator over the guidewire to make a tract in the subcutaneous tissue. A multihole pigtail or straight catheter is advanced over the wire into the pericardial space. Connect the distal end of the pigtail catheter to the 3-way stopcock and attach a 50 ml syringe and a drainage bag to the 3-way stopcock.
- Aspirate the fluid using a 50 ml syringe and empty it in the drainage bag attached to a 3-way stopcock.
- Send the pericardial fluid for biochemical, immunological, cytological, and microbiological examination.
- Aspirate till there is no or minimal fluid in the pericardial cavity under echocardiography and remove the pigtail catheter. Apply a dressing at the insertion site.
- If there is a chance of reaccumulation, secure the pigtail catheter in place using a 2-0 silk suture for subsequent drainage. Usually the pigtail catheter is removed soon after pericardiocentesis or when drainage has decreased to <50 ml every 24 h.
- Follow up echocardiogram to assess reaccumulation of fluid in the pericardial space needs to be performed.
- Plan for pericardial window or pericardiotomy if indicated.

Complications

- Cardiac arrhythmias
- Cardiac puncture
- Pneumothorax
- Coronary artery injury
- Peritoneal puncture
- Diaphragmatic, liver, stomach, or splenic injury
- Death

Balloon Pericardiotomy

Indications

- Palliative procedure for recurrent pericardial effusions

Contraindications

- Infectious etiology of pericardial effusion
- Major coagulation disorders
- Effusive-constrictive pericarditis
- Large left pleural effusion
- Advanced respiratory insufficiency
- History of pneumonectomy
- If pericardial effusion is loculated on TTE, surgical drainage may be required.

Equipment

- Local anesthetic
- Pericardiocentesis kit as detailed above
- ATLAS balloon 26 mm in size

Procedure

- Ensure good local anesthesia and analgesia is on board as the procedure is painful.
- First perform pericardiocentesis and evacuate at least 50 % of the pericardial fluid. Exchange for an Amplatz stiff wire over a 7F dilator and ensure its position in the pericardial space.
- Advance serial dilators (upto 14 F to create a good tract in the skin and subcutaneous tissue to allow for easy passage of the balloon) over the Amplatz stiff wire and then position the ATLAS® balloon (20 to 26 mm in diameter /30 to 40 mm in length) in the pericardium way beyond the entry point. A 60 cc syringe with 1:3 diluted contrast is used to inflate the balloon under fluoroscopic guidance. The balloon is partially inflated first to an atm of 2 and pulled back until you see the distal tip getting squeezed with formation of a waist. Pull back the balloon so that the waist is at the center of the balloon and centered across the inferior pericardial border in the AP or lateral view. The entire balloon should be under the skin. The balloon is then slowly inflated to its nominal pressure so that the waist disappears and the balloon is fully inflated (Figs. 29.2 and 29.3).
- Pericardial fluid may be blood stained following balloon pericardiotomy and a pigtail catheter may be reintroduced to drain the remaining fluid.
- Remove the deflated balloon and the guidewire. Apply occlusive sterile dressing at the operative site.

Fig. 29.2 Tight waist at the pericardium (*arrow*) on initial balloon inflation

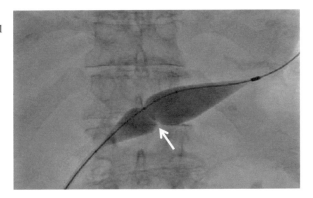

Fig. 29.3 Disappearance of the waist with full inflation of 26 mm/40 mm ATLAS balloon

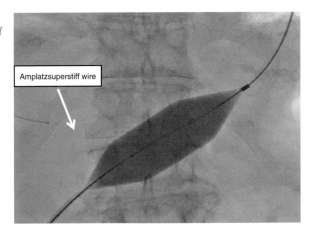

Post Procedure Monitor patient on a telemetry bed. Request for CXR and echocardiogram 24 h after the procedure. There will be left-sided pleural effusion due to pericardial drainage in the pleural space.

Recurrence Rate Mean survival of this group of patients is 3.6±3.8 months, and usually repeat balloon pericardiotomy is not required. 11 % recurrence rate at 54+/65 days was reported by an US percutaneous balloon pericardiotomy registry [1].

Reference

1. Ziskind AA, Palacios IF. Percutaneous balloon pericardiotomy for patients with pericardial effusion and tamponade. In: Topol EJ, editor. Textbook of interventional cardiology. 5th ed. Philadelphia: W.B. Saunders; 2007. p. 977–85.

Contrast-Induced Nephropathy Post Percutaneous Interventional Procedures

30

Anitha Rajamanickam and Annapoorna Kini

CIN is associated with increased morbidity and mortality, prolonged hospitalization, and increased healthcare costs. It is the third leading cause of hospital-acquired renal failure. The incidence of contrast-induced nephropathy (CIN) after cardiac catheterization reported in literature is 3–22 % [1–3]. CIN has been shown to be associated with additional morbidity, mortality, and increased healthcare costs [1, 2]. Although the mechanism for CIN is not understood, several mechanisms have been implicated in the pathogenesis of this complex phenomenon including direct cytotoxic effects of the contrast agents, ischemic injury due to renal vasoconstriction, decreases in renal medullary blood flow, auto- and paracrine effects (including adenosine, endothelin, and reactive oxygen species activity), oxidative stress, and cellular apoptosis [3]. Risk stratification prior to catheterization may help identify patients at high risk for CIN.

Definition

The National Kidney Foundation recommendation to create uniformity is to define acute kidney injury (AKI) including contrast-induced nephropathy (CIN) as any of the following:

- Rise in serum creatinine (SCr) by 0.3 mg/dl (26.5 l mol/l) $\leq$48 h
- Rise in SCr to 1.5 times from baseline $\leq$7 days
- Urine volume $\leq$0.5 ml/kg/h for 6 h [4].

A. Rajamanickam, MD (✉) • A. Kini, MD, MRCP, FACC
Department of Interventional Cardiology, Mount Sinai Hospital,
One Gustave Levy Place, Madison Avenue, New York, NY 10029, USA
e-mail: arajamanickam@gmail.com, Anitha.Rajamanickam@mountsinai.org;
Annapoorna.kini@mountsinai.org

© Springer-Verlag London 2014
A. Kini et al. (eds.), *Practical Manual of Interventional Cardiology*,
DOI 10.1007/978-1-4471-6581-1_30

Table 30.1 Risk factors for developing CIN

Modifiable risk factors	Nonmodifiable risk factors
First-generation hyperosmolar ionic contrast agents (rarely used)	Preexisting renal disease, CKD defined as a SCr >1.5 mg/dl or an eGFR of <60/ml/min
High contrast media dose	Diabetes
Nephrotoxic agents	Advanced age (>75)
Low hematocrit	Multiple myeloma
Low serum albumin (<35 g/L)	Renal transplant
Intra-aortic balloon pump	Acute myocardial infarction
Hypotension	LVEF <40 %
Hypovolemia	Advanced congestive heart failure and cardiogenic shock

However, the most commonly used definition of CIN in studies is 25 % increase in serum creatinine from baseline or 0.5 mg/dl (44 μmol/L) increase in absolute value $\leq$48–72 h after exposure to intravenous contrast that is not attributable to any other identifiable cause of renal failure. Usually creatinine levels peak at 3–5 days and usually return to normal in 2–4 weeks [4–6].

Identification of High-Risk Patients

Once CIN occurs, treatment is mainly supportive. Identification of high-risk patients for CIN is important as this will guide decision making. Higher-risk patients could then benefit from the therapies we currently employ to prevent this complication (Table 30.1 lists the risk factors for developing CIN).

- Risk assessment in all patients who are considered for cardiac catheterization.
- Substitute other imaging methods if feasible in high-risk patients.
- Two prior bedside calculators exist in the literature for calculating the estimated risk of CIN after a cardiac catheterization published by Mehran et al. and Baryholomew et al. [5, 6].

Prevention

The hallmark of therapy is prevention with aggressive volume expansion.

- Identify high-risk patients.
- Avoid nephrotoxins.
  - Nephrotoxins like metformin, nonsteroidal anti-inflammatory drugs (NSAID), aminoglycoside antibiotics, and immunosuppressive agents.
  - No conclusive data exists that holding chronic stable diuretics, angiotensin-converting enzyme inhibitors (ACEi), or angiotensin receptor blockers (ARB) is preventive.

Table 30.2 Preprocedural hydration

Start hydration with normal saline (0.9NS) 3 h prior to procedure if outpatient and 12 h prior if inpatient	
LVEF	For all patients but especially if SCr >1.3
>50	1–2 ml/kg/h
31–50	0.5 ml/kg/h
<30	0.3 ml/kg/h for 3 h in all patients

Table 30.3 Intraprocedural and postprocedural hydration

Continue hydration with normal saline (0.9 NS) during procedure and for 6–8 h post procedure if outpatient and 12 h if inpatient	
LVEF	For all patients but especially if SCr >1.3. If SCr <1.3, IVF can be given for a shorter duration with instructions for liberal discharge oral hydration
>50	1–2 ml/kg/h
<50	Measure LVEDP in the cath lab. Give a bolus of NS as per LVEDP
	<12: 500 cc
	12–18: 250 cc
	>18: No bolus
31–50	0.5 ml/kg/h
<30	0.3 ml/kg/h

- Volume supplementation: cornerstone of prevention of CIN.
  - Liberal oral hydration 24 h prior to the procedure.
  - Advise them to arrive at least 3 h prior to the procedure if outpatient.
  - Individualize treatment by symptoms and volume status.
  - In the absence of acute decompensated heart failure, follow Tables 30.2 and 30.3.
- *N*-Acetylcysteine: Though no conclusive data exists regarding its benefit, we prescribe it as it has no harmful side effects and is inexpensive.
  - 1,200 mg orally prior to and q 12 h×2 doses after cardiac catheterization
- Contrast
  - In high-risk patients, use isoosmolar (280–290 mOsm/kg) agents like iodixanol (Visipaque™) and hypo-osmolar agents like iopamidol (Optiray™). Avoid iohexol (Omnipaque™) and ioxaglate as these were associated with a higher incidence of CIN in trials [9].
  - Avoidance of hyper-osmolar (1,500–2,000 mOsm/kg) contrast media in all patients.
  - Limit the volume of RCM to as low as possible (preferably <100 ml).
- Use of smaller-caliber catheters.
- Avoid side-hole catheters.
- Avoid LV gram.
- Use "dry cine" and IVUS to guide stent sizing and placement.
- Prophylactic HD or hemofiltration has shown benefit in high-risk patients with creatinine clearance ≤30 ml/min or creatinine >2 mg/dl [7, 8].

- The data regarding the benefit of automated contrast injector systems has been conflicting.
- No conclusive data exists that statins, ascorbic acid, prostaglandin E1, post-procedure diuretics, mannitol, atrial natriuretic peptide, dopamine, calcium channel blockers, theophylline, and fenoldopam are preventive.

Post-procedure Monitoring

- Check SCr >24 h and <72 h post RCM exposure.
- Hydration with normal saline 0.9 NS at 1–1.5 mg/kg/h for 12 h in high-risk patients to maintain urine output (150 ml/h if achievable).
- The use of sodium bicarbonate solutions may allow shorter supplementation periods.
- Hold all nephrotoxins until renal function returns to baseline.

Treatment

- Evaluate for other causes of AKI.
- Hold all nephrotoxins.
- HD if patient is oliguric or anuric as per nephrology recommendations.
- Patient may be discharged with close outpatient monitoring once the SCr starts returning down towards normal baseline levels.
- Outpatient follow-up with repeat SCr in 2–3 days.
- The identification of high-risk individuals, aggressive volume repletion, avoidance of concurrent nephrotoxins, the use of low-volume hypo-osmolar or iso-osmolar RCM, and close post-procedure follow-up are vital in the prevention of CIN.

References

1. Rihal CS, Textor SC, Grill DE, et al. Incidence and prognostic importance of acute renal failure after percutaneous coronary intervention. Circulation. 2002;105(19):2259–64.
2. McCullough PA, Wolyn R, Rocher LL, Levin RN, O'Neill WW. Acute renal failure after coronary intervention: incidence, risk factors, and relationship to mortality. Am J Med. 1997;103(5):368–75.
3. Deek H, Newton P, Sheerin N, Noureddine S, Davidson PM. Contrast media induced nephropathy: a literature review of the available evidence and recommendations for practice. Aust Crit Care. 2014;pii:S1036-7314(13)00266-X. doi:10.1016/j.aucc.2013.12.002. [Epub ahead of print] PubMed PMID: 24461960.
4. Kidney Disease: Improving Global Outcomes (KDIGO) Acute Kidney Injury Work Group. KDIGO clinical practice guideline for acute kidney injury. Kidney Int Suppl. 2012;2:1–138.
5. Mehran R, Aymong ED, Nikolsky E, et al. A simple risk score for prediction of contrast-induced nephropathy after percutaneous coronary intervention: development and initial validation. J Am Coll Cardiol. 2004;44(7):1393–9.

6. Bartholomew BA, Harjai KJ, Dukkipati S, et al. Impact of nephropathy after percutaneous coronary intervention and a method for risk stratification. Am J Cardiol. 2004;93(12):1515–9.
7. Marenzi G, Lauri G, Campodonico J, Marana I, Assanelli E, De Metrio M, Grazi M, Veglia F, Fabbiocchi F, Montorsi P, Bartorelli AL. Comparison of two hemofiltration protocols for prevention of contrast-induced nephropathy in high-risk patients. Am J Med. 2006;119(2):155–62. PubMed PMID: 16443418.
8. Marenzi G, Bartorelli AL. Hemofiltration in the prevention of radiocontrast agent induced nephropathy. Minerva Anestesiol. 2004;70(4):189–91. PubMed PMID: 15173694.

Made in United States
Cleveland, OH
10 December 2024

11648223R00190